AGING AND THE BRAIN

ADVANCES IN BEHAVIORAL BIOLOGY

AGING AND THE BRAIN

The Proceedings of the Fifth Annual Symposium held at
the Texas Research Institute of Mental Sciences in Houston,
October 1971

Edited by
Charles M. Gaitz

Chief, Gerontology Research Section
Texas Research Institute of Mental Sciences
Houston, Texas

ℚ PLENUM PRESS • NEW YORK–LONDON • 1972

First Printing — May 1972
Second Printing — January 1976

Annual symposia on research in behavioral biology have been held at the Texas Research Institute of Mental Sciences since 1967. The proceedings of the first three—*Congenital Mental Retardation, Drug Dependence,* and *Biological Aspects of Alcohol*—were published by the University of Texas Press, Austin, Texas.

Library of Congress Catalog Card Number 72-77227

ISBN 0-306-37903-1

© 1972 Plenum Press, New York
A Division of Plenum Publishing Corporation
227 West 17th Street, New York, N.Y. 10011

United Kingdom edition published by Plenum Press, London
A Division of Plenum Publishing Company, Ltd.
Davis House (4th Floor), 8 Scrubs Lane, Harlesden, London, NW10
6SE, England

Preface

This volume contains the proceedings of the fifth annual symposium held October 1971 at the Texas Research Institute of Mental Sciences in Houston.

We are grateful to Curtin Scientific Company, Fisher Scientific Company, Geigy Pharmaceuticals, The Gerontological Society, ICN Bentex Pharmaceutical Company, Ives Laboratories, Knoll Pharmaceutical Company, Merck Sharp & Dohme Postgraduate Program, The Moody Foundation, The Pauline Sterne Wolff Memorial Home, Pfizer Laboratories, Roche Laboratories, Sandoz Pharmaceuticals, Schering Corporation, and E.R. Squibb & Sons for their generous financial support of the symposium.

Special thanks to Dr. William M. McIsaac, director of Texas Research Institute, for his guidance of the symposium series, and to administrator Frank J. Womack and his staff for organizational support. To Drs. Neil R. Burch, James L. Claghorn, Beng T. Ho, Robert J. Johnson, and Joseph C. Schoolar, heads of Institute research departments, thanks for their contribution in chairing symposium sessions. To Lore Feldman, who claims all typographical errors, credit for skillful copy editing of the manuscript. Typesetting was done by Gee Lindblom of the medical illustration and audiovisual education department at Baylor College of Medicine.

Charles M. Gaitz

Contributors

Paul E. Baer, Ph.D.
    Professor, Department of Psychiatry, Baylor College of Medicine, Houston, Texas

Arthur L. Benton, Ph.D.
    Professor of Neurology and Psychology, University of Iowa, Iowa City, Iowa

James E. Birren, Ph.D.
    Director, Gerontology Center, University of Southern California, Los Angeles, California

Ewald W. Busse, M.D.
    J.P. Gibbons Professor of Psychiatry and Chairman, Department of Psychiatry, Duke University College of Medicine, Durham, North Carolina

Carl Eisdorfer, Ph.D., M.D.
    Professor of Psychiatry; Professor and Head, Division of Medical Psychology; Director, Center for the Study of Aging and Human Development, Duke University Medical Center, Durham, North Carolina

William S. Fields, M.D.
    Professor of Neurology, The University of Texas Medical School at Houston, Houston, Texas

Joseph M. Foley, M.D., Sc.D.
    Professor of Neurology, Case Western Reserve University, Cleveland, Ohio

Charles M. Gaitz, M.D.
    Chief, Gerontology Research Section, Texas Research Institute of Mental Sciences, Houston, Texas

Alvin I. Goldfarb, M.D.
    Associate Clinical Professor of Psychiatry, Mount Sinai School of Medicine of the City University of New York, New York

Raymond Harris, M.D.
  Clinical Assistant Professor of Medicine, Albany Medical College; Chief, Subdepartment of Cardiovascular Medicine, St. Peter's Hospital, Albany, New York

David W.K. Kay, M.D.
  Consultant in Psychiatry, Royal Victoria Infirmary; Honorary Lecturer in Psychiatry, University of Newcastle upon Tyne, Newcastle upon Tyne, United Kingdom

Heinz E. Lehmann, M.D.
  Professor and Chairman, Department of Psychiatry, McGill University; Director of Medical Education and Research, Douglas Hospital, Verdun, Quebec, Canada

Nathan Malamud, M.D.
  Professor of Neuropathology, University of California, San Francisco; Chief, Neuropathology Service, Langley Porter Neuropsychiatric Institute, San Francisco, California

Walter D. Obrist, Ph.D.
  Professor of Medical Psychology, Duke University Medical Center, Durham, North Carolina

J. Mark Ordy, Ph.D.
  Professor, Department of Psychology, Northern Illinois University, DeKalb, Illinois

Thaddeus Samorajski, Ph.D.
  Director, Laboratory of Neurochemistry, Cleveland Psychiatric Institute; Assistant Clinical Professor, Experimental Neuropathology, Case Western Reserve University, Cleveland, Ohio

Robert D. Terry, M.D.
  Professor and Chairman, Department of Pathology, Albert Einstein College of Medicine, The Bronx, New York

Maurice W. Van Allen, M.D.
  Professor of Neurology and Director, Neurosensory Center, University of Iowa, Iowa City, Iowa

Jack Weinberg, M.D.
  Professor of Psychiatry, Abraham Lincoln School of Medicine, University of Illinois, and Clinical Director, Illinois State Psychiatric Institute, Chicago, Illinois

Henryk M. Wiśniewski, M.D., Ph.D.
  Associate Professor of Pathology, Albert Einstein College of Medicine, The Bronx, New York; Career Scientist of the Health Research Council of the City of New York

Contents

Psychological and Epidemiological Aspects

Chemical and Pathological Aspects

Physiological and Diagnostic Aspects

Clinical Aspects

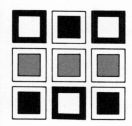

Prologue

Charles M. Gaitz, M.D.

Gerontology Research Section
Texas Research Institute of Mental Sciences
Houston, Texas

Much anxiety is expressed in our day about the declining quality of life and the dehumanizing effects of startling advances in technology, even of those in biology and medicine. These worries find their saddest confirmation in the existence of the elderly people in our society, whose numbers are increasing, whose lives have been lengthened and, almost correspondingly, robbed of content and purpose. As Leon R. Kass said recently of old people, "we have learned how to increase their years, but we have not learned how to help them enjoy their days" (*Science* November 19, 1971). Knowing how to prolong life, we do not know what to do with it. Or, knowing how to enrich living, we are unwilling or unable to transform our understanding into practice.

This, basically, was the reason for the symposium we held on Aging and the Brain. We luckily attracted many of the outstanding experts in a number of disciplines concerned with the care of elderly persons. Our purpose was and is to identify better ways of distributing and delivering health care and to back up these systems with a deeper knowledge, both social and scientific, that will lead to prevention and amelioration of the diseases and maladaptions of aging.

Our specific concern is the care of the elderly mentally ill. We want to go beyond the highly visible issues—state hospital versus nursing home, for example—because treatment in the finest medical institutions leaves much to be desired. To do this, we must first clarify the critical issues in prevention and treatment of mental illness in aged persons and pinpoint the problems and obstacles that have prevented us, so far, from doing a better job. We need a "baseline," a description of where we are now: what we are reasonably certain are the changes that occur with aging, particularly as they relate to brain functions. We must examine the diagnostic tools we have, their limitations, the risks involved in their use, and to review and appraise the treatment modalities available.

1

All of us admit that most treatment programs are pragmatic, and that a rational basis, one underpinned by knowledge of the etiology of the condition being treated, is needed. Some therapists would argue that any theoretical formulation, even a faulty one, has value as a frame of reference; it is reassuring and gives therapists confidence in what they do. But the closer we come to the "truth" in our theoretical formulations, the more likely we are to prescribe appropriately. This principle applies when we are concerned with etiology of disease, mechanism of action of a therapeutic agent, or with altering the environment in which treatment is undertaken. Value judgments will always be made in planning treatment programs. But, logically, the more we know about cause-and-effect relationships, the more likely we are to initiate treatment programs that have some promise of success.

Concepts are changing rapidly. More and more psychiatric disorders, for example, are being classified as "organic" (not that classification is proof); the alcoholic psychoses are classified as organic disorders in the latest diagnostic manual of the American Psychiatric Association, and other disorders may be so classified in the future.

The fact is, however, that transfer of a disorder from one category to another—from one basket to another—will not help clinicians substantively. Treatment will improve only as we learn more about etiology and can achieve a better fit between etiology, pathology, and treatment modalities.

We began the symposium with the realization that we would ask questions that probably could not be answered at our present level of understanding, no matter how knowledgeable our assembly of experts. Our concerns were numerous and broad. We were concerned with such issues as the relationship of aging to the progression of neurotic and psychotic disorders and the long-term effects of treatment, even of psychoanalysis, on the character structure of elderly persons. We wondered whether there is a relationship between the symptomatology of organic brain syndrome and etiology. Would it be possible to delineate common factors that produce a delirium when the etiology appears to be as varied as the toxicity of drugs or alcohol, a postoperative psychosis, uremia, congestive heart failure, or respiratory disease? Does chronological age affect the pharmacology of psychotropic drugs? In the light of present knowledge, can we continue to think of symptoms as "functional" or "organic"? And if this frame of reference is not satisfactory, what alternative do we have? What more can we learn about the relationship of mental and physical health? How useful are current diagnostic techniques? How can we more accurately predict prognosis? What better criteria can be established for the effectiveness of the many recommended agents and medical regimens? Conceivably, too, organic brain syndrome is so broad a concept as to have little meaning, and yet there is no better description for the way organic changes in the brain substance are associated with behavioral changes.

The "answers"—either for theoretical formulations or for treatment—are not likely to come from one single professional discipline, but from a collaboration and the pooling of information by many. The diseases that concern us have their origin in many factors.

This is the thesis on which the symposium on Aging and the Brain was planned. We gathered representatives from psychology, pathology, pharmacology, and chemistry, and clinicians in neurology, psychiatry, and internal medicine. Having more rational and effective methods of prevention and treatment as our objective, we realized gaps in knowledge had to be filled before this could be achieved. We therefore asked the speakers at the symposium to direct their presentations to persons in other disciplines, to bring them up to date on current status, and to present their material in a way that would lend itself to integration with data from other disciplines. This approach has certain advantages and some disadvantages as well. This book, obviously, cannot provide a thorough review of each topic, but we believe it is a provocative and stimulating sample of many.

We arbitrarily limited our areas of concern. Competent investigators have demonstrated the influences on behavior of sociological, social, and economic factors, but we gave these little attention. Instead, our emphasis was on exploring the behavior described as organic brain syndrome, relating it to our current knowledge of anatomic, physiologic, and pathologic changes in the brain, and drawing conclusions from such relationships that are relevant to understanding the behavioral changes associated with altered functions of the aging brain.

We attempted to differentiate "normal" and "abnormal" aging processes. That such differentiation should be possible is logical, but the conceptual problems in defining normality—in terms of the neurobiological and neuropathological changes in aged persons—are very complex. One may take the position that decline in function is inevitably associated with aging and therefore not abnormal, and that the rate of change varies from individual to individual. Another possible position is that any diminution of function is evidence of the presence and processes of disease and not attributable to chronological aging at all. Then, too, normality and abnormality may be conceptualized as a matter of degree, relating, for example, to the number of cells lost with aging, or the extent of the areas of damage. Conceptions of normal and abnormal aging are discussed in some of the papers, but the answers are still not clear.

It is with such matters that we were concerned in this symposium.

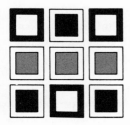

**Cognitive Changes in Aging:
Competence and Incompetence**

Paul E. Baer, Ph.D.

Department of Psychiatry, Baylor College of Medicine
Houston, Texas

The mental infirmities of old age are commonly accorded a close second in inevitability after death and taxes. What has been taken virtually as a truism, that persons deteriorate psychologically as they become older, today seems less a simple truth. This discussion will be devoted to a modest polemic, the thesis that the cognitive capabilities the elderly retain should be understood as well as the capabilities they lose.

To advance this thesis, first there will be commentary on views and observations that suggest the need for emphasis on the capacities of the aged, as well as on their incapacities. Second will be an attempt at preliminary formulation of a theoretical position that is intended to accommodate not only decline, but the capabilities of the aged as well. Third I shall review several studies selected to illustrate that certain research findings support the plausibility of the theoretical position to be proposed. The term cognitive is used in a broad, descriptive sense. Furthermore, this approach is not meant to diminish in any way the importance of understanding mental deficits in the elderly.

The level of performance among elderly persons has been shown to be importantly influenced by factors other than age, namely health, education, intelligence, and vocational background. Certain functions, such as psychomotor speed, are particularly susceptible to aging effects, as opposed to others that are less vulnerable. There may well be a kind of interplay, possibly a synergism, among various kinds of functions. Consequently, observed impairment in one cognitive function may not simply reflect failure of that particular function, but that of another underlying, contributing or correlated function that is a component in the cognitive performance under consideration. Such impressions are readily generated when one reviews recent work concerning the role of time and speed in the performance of the elderly, the details of learning and recall processes, and elements of judgment and decision-making. Of

5

additional importance are a number of methodologic issues involving sampling, the characteristics of the elderly persons under study, and the nature of the context in which research is conducted, for these may seriously affect the extent to which cognitive impairments are demonstrated.

Although studies typically show a decline in cognitive functions among the elderly, these declines are not observed universally. There have been instances, in fact, in which it was found that young and old persons performed recall tasks equally well (e.g., Hulicka and Weiss 1965; Keevil-Rogers and Schnore 1969). This is especially the case in the performance of selected aging samples in whom health, education, socioeconomic background, and current status are controlled. Declines may be a function, for example, of ill health or disuse of intellectual capabilities rather than of old age.

To further illustrate this point, results of an unpublished study conducted at the Texas Research Institute of Mental Sciences may be cited. We examined the performance of two groups of elderly individuals in good health, all over the age of 60, with one group averaging 65 and the other 75 years of age. In addition, two other comparably aged groups were assessed, and these were comprised of patients institutionalized for chronic brain syndrome associated with aging. The battery of tests included procedures for assessing verbal and motor performance, sensory and perceptual abilities, language functions, memory and higher cognitive functions. The first two groups of individuals, all of whom lived in the community and were able to maintain themselves to the extent of moving freely about the city, showed no age changes in performance. The two groups of impaired individuals, however, showed a number of significant declines for the older compared to the younger group. The "normal" groups, of course, performed far better than the institutionalized groups. Of further interest was the finding that for the "normal" groups there was a significant correlation in performance to the extent to which the individuals had been educated earlier in their lives. This finding also suggests a comment on the role of sampling in research with older populations. One reason the older "normal" sample did not show decline in performance may have been that, as individuals grow older and show signs of deterioration with increasing age, they become lost to the pool of "normal" persons because they no longer can meet the criteria for membership in that group. If they are moderately ill they may be confined to their homes; if they become sufficiently ill they may become institutionalized. This implies that there may be a measurable minimal level of health and performance that is necessary for the elderly individual to remain in the community.

It is important to consider, further, that the cognitive performance of aged persons can be experimentally manipulated, and that under certain conditions their performance can be enhanced. It has also been established that the rate of decline varies for different abilities, and that certain abilities, such as those measured by vocabulary tests, resist decline and may grow with age. With regard to the circumstances under which the cognitive functions of the elderly are studied, the degree of arousal generated in a testing or experimental session, in terms of interest or in terms of anxiety, may have significant bearing on performance. For the elderly, possibly much more than for younger persons, there is a critical question concerning the degree of correspondence between what is assessed in the laboratory and problem-solving in the natural environment.

Such issues may be fruitfully reconsidered in the perspective of a proposed theoretical statement concerned with perceptual cognitive functions in aging. An attempt at devising the rudiments of such a statement seems timely, if only for heuristic purposes, first because the field seems characterized by a transitional status, second to parallel theoretical developments at the biological level, and third to offer avenues for construction of hypotheses consistent with emerging research trends.

The current literature reveals no systematic efforts geared to formulation of theory for cognitive processes and aging (Busse 1969). This limitation does not mean that current research is exclusively empirical. On the contrary, viable controversial theoretical positions are being investigated, such as attempts to account for memory deficits by interference, disuse, or inadequate storage. The type of model aimed for should have scope for such explanations of specific functions. A more general theoretical approach that has enjoyed support for some time is one that accounts for aging effects from a developmental standpoint. It posits that developmental processes of growth, as initially observed in childhood, are also applicable for the understanding of changes at the other polar end of the life span. If the position to be proposed undergoes sufficient elaboration, the results should clarify whether it can be subsumed under a more general developmental theory or not.

Much current work on aging effects remains centered on the decline of cognitive functions in the elderly organism. In fact, one is left with a general impression that research on aging inherently represents a psychology of decline and deficit. The aura of aging viewed as a pathogenic process is difficult to dispel. Problems in interpretation arise when the studies do not provide results consistent with expectations of decline, as is sometimes the case. These unpredicted negative outcomes are subject to question, especially in the absence of a system or framework readily available for understanding them.

It should be noted that a strict concern with decline or deficit in a quantitative sense also masks the possibility that qualitative changes may occur. Such qualitative changes may or may not be interpreted as representing decline. They may represent attempts of the older individual to adjust or cope. The approach of an older person to problem-solving may involve a qualitatively different set than that of a younger individual. The older person, for example, may deal with problems in a less abstract fashion.

With reference to the problem of research on intervention in processes of aging, Comfort (1970) has cogently described built-in limits for the human life span. Better health care and improved nutrition have yielded lower mortality rates at younger ages but have not extended the life span. A next major effort in biological aging research requires study of the genetic code as it relates to control of the life span. A model designed to promote intervention-oriented research with respect to cognitive functions seems to be particularly congenial to developments in biological research. In any event, emphasis on the preservation and enhancement of cognitive processes in aging has social value in its own right.

The model to be proposed can be visualized in a framework analogous to one described by Meerloo (1970) in cybernetic terms. Its requirements are that it concern measurable functions, that it predict competence as well as incompetence, that it deal with aging as a complex process not exclusively involving decline, and that it identify and describe conditions other than aging which alter functions that are actually or potentially related to aging. According to such a model, aging is seen as a process in which a functioning, self-correcting system with reserve capacity makes progressively increasing demands both on auto-regulation and reserve capacity.

In accord with this proposition, the level of a cognitive function is defined as a product of capability in a specific function and conditions that affect the utilization of that capability. Such conditions may be internal or external to the organism. In either case they may facilitate or impede use of the capability in question.

Applied to the aging human organism, the model suggests that cognitive processes can be viewed as progressively declining, but that the decline is observed only in contexts that allow decline. Conversely, there may be other contexts in which decline is not observed. The aging organism is seen as adaptively seeking situations and contexts that minimize the degree of decline. The extent of decline in a particular function, the development and availability of compensatory internal capabilities or strategies, the status of environmental demands, and the opportunity to control the environment are all ingredients in producing the level of functioning.

In terms of this formulation, capability and the extent of decline can not be directly observed but must be inferred from performance. It is possible, however, to affect performance by enhancing compensatory processes, for example by drugs or by training. Moreover, by manipulating the context in which cognitive performance is assessed, a number of processes may be activated to either supress or potentiate performance. Among them are those that respond to reinforcement and those concerned with stress. In general, performance level is expected to reflect the complex interplay of capability and the organism's effort to moderate deficits. These efforts may themselves contribute to decline rather than to enhancement because of misconceptions and judgmental failures. The self-regulatory mechanisms can themselves become impaired.

In order to ascertain the potential utility of the model that has been briefly described, a few studies from the literature have been chosen to exemplify how the outcomes of these studies conform with the theoretical position. It is not possible to check the model in detail, and at this early stage the level of sophistication of the examples may be somewhat low. One of the points made in this argument was that there may be an inherent limit on certain capacities associated with aging, but that the performance involving that capacity could be shown to be affected by various factors. The more clearly the limits of a particular capacity can be demonstrated, the better the case can be made for identifying and describing the conditions that produce improved performance. Thus, a critical task in developing the model would be to isolate the ingredients of performance decrement so that those components concerned with capacity can be distinguished from those more subject to control. In the present instance, speed of response and the role of time in performance have been chosen for illustrative purposes. As will be seen in a number of interesting ways, recent research has focused on time and on speed of response as a central element in perceptual cognitive performance in aging.

Psychomotor slowing, whether observed in simple or choice reaction time experiments, or in more complex problem-solving situations, is a ubiquitous accompaniment of aging. Its basis, to a relatively minor extent, is impulse transmission velocity and motor speed and, to a much larger extent, the central processes conjectured to involve, among other possibilities, retarded intercellular transfer or reduction in neural excitability. Despite the implication that, essentially, slowing has a nonpsychological core, reduced response speed associated with aging varies with psychological factors. Differences in speed of performance between groups of elderly individuals have been demonstrated in a number of ways, and they exemplify how reaction time performance in aging may be enhanced.

In the case of simple reaction time, a motor act, usually the lifting of a finger from a microswitch or a telegraph key, is timed for the latency of its occurrence following an imperative signal, or signal to act. Preparation for the imperative signal and motor act has important bearing on the speed of response. In many studies the imperative signal is preceded by a preparatory or alerting signal, which the imperative signal follows after varying time periods ranging from one-half second to 15 seconds or longer, in regular or irregular sequence. Botwinick and Thompson (1967) showed that over a series of repeated occasions of a simple reaction time task, the speed of response of elderly subjects improved when the preparatory intervals were of the same duration, that is, in regular sequence. Improvement with practice was noted particularly for a brief one-half second preparatory interval, but lengthing this interval to as long as 15 seconds did not assist the elderly in reducing reaction time.

It is of interest to contrast this finding with results reported for choice reaction time. In that situation two or more responses are possible, and each response is linked to its own imperative signal. Here, again, it has been shown that reaction time improves with practice. Talland (1964) showed that reaction time of elderly persons improved when the preparatory interval was lengthened to 4 seconds, as compared to shorter preparatory intervals. In a somewhat more complex situation, Rabbitt (1964) showed that elderly persons are able to retain response speed levels whether they are given information to assist them in responding or not. Given misleading information, however, their reaction times became retarded considerably more than that of younger subjects. Finally, it should come as no surprise that the status of health of the elderly has bearing on reaction time. With respect to the model, the point is that response speed of elderly individuals can increase with practice, and that under some conditions, older persons can take good advantage of the opportunity for preparation to respond. Information is an important element in the response speed of the elderly.

The implications of slowing pose a critical question. Does slowing have significance for other functions in which speed of response, or time available for responding, is a factor? Rabbitt and Birren (1967) conducted an experiment in which regular sequences of visual signals were presented to the subjects, who responded by rapidly touching switches mounted under the signals. Occasionally another light was flashed that did not fit the regular sequence. One type of error that occurred involved continued responding in the sequence despite interruptions in the sequence of signals. Older subjects responded more slowly than younger subjects but made fewer errors of this type. The data also suggested that when the elderly did commit continuation errors, their response speed on the preceding regular sequence was faster and more in the range of the response speed of the younger subjects. The investigators proposed that the extended reaction times of the elderly were functional in that they assisted the elderly in maintaining a degree of efficiency.

The data also yielded the conclusion that the quality of the performance of the elderly individuals differed from that of the younger ones. The younger subjects learned to respond to sequences in which the signals were presented, but the older subjects seemed to respond to the signals in a segmented manner, treating each signal as a single instance for responding. The tendency of the older individuals not to make continuation errors can be understood in the context of their not responding to a sequential system.

From another prespective, research on verbal learning and memory has shown, apart from the fact that the extent of verbal learning and recall can be manipulated for the elderly, that the amount of time available for the task has important bearing on the level of performance. In order to control various factors operative in verbal learning, stimulus words or nonmeaningful materials are presented to the subjects in a carefully timed method, which can call for specified exposure times, specified response times, and specified interval durations between the presentations of successive words. In serial learning a list of words is presented one at a time, and the subject is asked to indicate the next word in the list. Eisdorfer (1968) showed that elderly subjects make fewer omission errors; that is, they fail to respond less often as exposure and response times are extended. Commission errors, those involving wrong responses, are not affected.

In paired associate learning, pairs of words are systematically presented, one word of a pair first, and the subject is asked to indicate the associated word. Arenberg (1965) reported that the less rapid the rate at which material is presented and the more time allowed for responding, especially if there is unlimited time, the better older persons learn. Factors other than time, such as ease of task, availability of cues, and augmented sensory input, have also been identified as supporting verbal learning and performance of elderly subjects.

An example of particular interest concerns a study of the role of learning in the investigation of memory. In the study of memory, the question generally arises whether or not the subject's level of recall is a consequence of the extent to which he has learned the material to be remembered. Consequently, in an experimental setting, subjects who are to be examined for rate of recall are first given opportunities to learn the material. Efforts are made to control the degree of learning. This distinction between learning and memory is particularly applicable to study of memory in aged individuals, who are so often deficient in recall. Hulicka and Weiss (1965) found that when elderly subjects were permitted to learn paired associates to a criterion, they required many more trials than did younger subjects. However, when their memory for the paired associates was examined after they had learned the material to criterion, their recall was no worse than that of younger subjects. It should be added that this kind of finding is somewhat controversial because there is also evidence to the contrary. For present purposes, however, the fact that such an outcome can occur is sufficient to make the point that for these older subjects, compensatory processes associated with learning seemed to be importantly involved in recall.

A number of possibilities have been considered to account for the impaired performance of the elderly when the element of time is important. It has been contended, for example, that older individuals are more cautious, and delay or inhibit performance to maximize accuracy. Experimental tasks may be inappropriate for the elderly, who are no longer familiar with or concerned with tests and assessment of performance. Disinterest, resentment, or disruptive anxiety may occur. Research has been conducted in which the performance of the older person does not involve skill, but primarily cautiousness and decision-making. To illustrate the role of response time in such a situation and to demonstrate performance of older subjects contrasted to younger subjects, a dissertation done by Miriam Robins (1969) in our laboratory will be briefly described.

Robins' procedure had the advantage, apart from not demanding skill, of having a high degree of familiarity for a group of older subjects living in the community, aged 65 or above. A circular bingo cage was used in which there were 36 balls, each inscribed with a number from 2 to 12. By varying the number of balls marked with different digits, it was possible to achieve correspondence with the chance events of two fair dice, when the cage was rotated and a ball was ejected. Forty elderly subjects, and an equal number of college-aged subjects, were instructed to bet one of four possible amounts on one of seven lettered positions, each position indicating a specified probability for winning in a range from two chances in three to one chance in 18. If the subject won, he was paid off according to the matrix that was always in view and had been carefully explained. There were 30 trials, each involving a bet and a pay-off. Half of each group of 40 subjects had chips worth cash. The response latency was recorded for decision to bet, which the subject indicated by placing a chip on a probability marker. It was ascertained that all subjects understood the procedure. For present purposes it is of interest to note that overall, older patients responded much more slowly than younger subjects; that is, they took more time to decide probability choice and to bet. The older subjects chose less risky probabilities than did the younger subjects, not to a substantial degree, but enough to assure them more wins. On the other hand, there was no difference between old and young in the amounts bet, and when bet and probability choices were combined in a pay-off measure, the aged groups did not differ from the young groups. Decisions made after instances of winning or losing were examined separately. All groups, old and young alike, shifted choice of probability upward after losing and downward after winning. Both young and old groups had shorter latencies of response after losing than after winning. These data are cited here primarily to illustrate a situation in which the slowed response of the elderly in a nonskill situation was not associated with inappropriateness of response, in the sense of contrast with a younger sample. Further, and perhaps more importantly, it was demonstrated that older persons performed adaptively and adjusted their behavior flexibly to the contingencies of the situation, irrespective of the time required to act.

In this discussion, the issue of cognitive competence in the elderly has not been approached in terms of the central concern of this symposium, namely, the status of the elderly person's brain. For present purposes, senescence and senility are to be distinguished, a distinction that is practically useful. A case in point is the investigation of the role of the brain in aging effects among healthy older individuals. Maintaining the position that aging and brain damage are not identical allows application of conceptual schemes of the type outlined. Brain damage can be conceptualized as one of a number of possible individual difference variables that can be studied in relation to aging.

To summarize, the preliminary theoretical proposition and the data described were meant to draw attention to the need to broaden the perspectives of research on cognitive processes in aging. Substantial progress has been made in the understanding of deficiencies and decline in cognitive performance of elderly persons. The time seems right to add an additional dimension to our efforts to understand how elderly persons perform. What is now needed are more studies examining the competence of older persons. In particular, an attitude emphasizing competence as well as incompetence could generate research on a problem about which little is known, namely, the effects of social reinforcement on the performance of the elderly. When one examines the social fabric in more general terms, it is apparent that society provides relatively few rewards for competence in the aged. On the contrary, at best, the social atmosphere is one of relative disregard, or nonreward. Perhaps an extended view in research can be the forerunner of a more general change in social attitudes toward the aged.

References

Arenberg, D. 1965. Anticipation interval and age differences in verbal learning. *J. Abnorm. Psychol.* 70:419.

Botwinick, J., and Thompson, L.W. 1967. Practice of speeded response in relation to age, sex and set. *J. Geront.* 22:72.

Busse, E.W. 1969. Theories of aging. In *Behavior and Adaptation in Late Life.* E.W. Busse and E. Pfeiffer (eds.). Boston: Little Brown, p. 11.

Comfort, A. 1970. Biological theories of aging. *Hum. Develop.* 13:127.

Eisdorfer, C. 1968. Arousal and performance: Experiments in verbal learning and a tentative theory. In *Human Aging and Behavior.* G.A. Talland (ed.). New York: Academic Press, p. 189.

Hulicka, I.M., and Weiss, R.L. 1965. Age differences in retention as a function of learning. *J. Consult. Psychol.* 29:125.

Keevil-Rogers, P., and Schnore, M.M. 1969. Short-term memory as a function of age in persons of above average intelligence. *J. Geront.* 24:184.

Meerloo, J.A. 1970. The cybernoses of the aged — the failure of self-regulating mechanisms. *J. Amer. Geriat. Soc.* 18:692.

Rabbitt, P.M. 1964. Set and age in a choice-response task. *J. Geront.* 19:301.

Rabbitt, P.M., and Birren, J.E. 1967. Age and responses to sequences of repetitive and interruptive signals. *J. Geront.* 22:143.

Robins, M.R. Risk taking as a function of age, monetary incentive, and gain or loss. Unpublished doctoral dissertation, University of Houston, 1969.

Talland, G.A. 1964. The effect of warning signals on reaction time in youth and old age. *J. Geront.* 19:31.

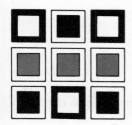

Epidemiological Aspects of Organic Brain Disease in the Aged

D.W.K. Kay, M.D.

Royal Victoria Infirmary and
University of Newcastle upon Tyne
Newcastle upon Tyne, England

Demographic Aspects

The epidemiology of the organic brain syndromes that occur in old age merits our attention today for two main reasons. In the first place, many more people are surviving into old age, and secondly, old people are particularly prone to mental disorder. Of all mental and physical handicaps that afflict the aged, the chronic brain syndromes are among the most disabling and make the heaviest demands on the resources of the state and the family. In Britain, since the beginning of the century, the absolute number of those aged 65 and over has increased four-fold, and those aged over 85 have increased seven-fold. Similar changes have occurred elsewhere, and population projections show that the very old will for a time continue to increase at a faster rate than other age groups. The fall in the birth rate, which has increased the proportion of the old to the young in many countries, is now reaching its full effect in some places, but the fall in mortality among the young will continue, and spread, and cause a permanent aging of populations. If and when the killing diseases of middle and later life are brought under control, there will be a further increase of the old and very old. Social changes such as the migration of the young in search of work, or indeed any social movements that tend to detach the younger from the older generations, will accentuate the isolation of the aged and throw the responsibility for their care more and more onto the state and other agencies.

Clinical Aspects

The organic mental syndromes, as I would prefer to call them, arise from structural changes in the brain or from interference with its function from any cause. They may be mild or severe, but they have in common the following basic features: (1) impairment of memory, particularly the registration of on-going events; (2) impairment of intellectual

15

function, such as comprehension, calculation, and learning; and (3) disorientation for place and time. Not all these features need be present to the same degree and when, for example, amnesia or "parietal lobe" symptoms are particularly prominent, they have localizing significance. There are, however, two main types of brain syndrome, and it is essential to distinguish between them (Table 1). The *acute and subacute syndromes* are characterized by clouding of consciousness, causing confusion or delirium, and are potentially reversible states. The *chronic syndromes* are, in the aged, usually due to widespread destructive or degenerative processes and are usually progressive.

The details of the clinical picture in acute and subacute brain syndromes are determined by the specific cause, which may be an acute lesion (e.g., traumatic or vascular) in the brain itself. In a large group of cases, however, there is no structural damage to the brain, and the disturbance is due to systemic illness such as cardiac failure, acute or chronic respiratory disease, surgical operations, dehydration and electrolyte disturbances, anemias, malignant disease, or to intoxications or vitamin and nutritional deficiencies. Clouding of consciousness is a sign of an unstable state, and so long as it exists a change either for better or for worse (coma and death) can be anticipated. With recovery the mental state returns as a rule to its previous level, which may be impaired if there is a chronic brain syndrome, but may be fully normal in previously normal people.

In the chronic syndromes the level of mental function is reduced, not merely below the person's own previous level, but below the level of any normal person. It is not a matter, from the clinician's point of view, simply of becoming more stupid, slow, and forgetful, but of qualitative departures from normal mental function. This is what is usually meant by the term "dementia," which implies a disorganization of everyday behavior. Lesser degrees of mental impairment and specific defects will, of course, also be encountered and may be reported as "mild dementia" or "mild mental deterioration," a category that is ill-defined clinically and probably heterogeneous. The fact that it exists, however, is of interest from several points of view.

Emotional disturbances, changes in mood, and psychotic features such as delusions and hallucinations are frequent in brain syndromes, but the traditional notion that *all* forms of mental illness arising in old age are basically due to underlying cerebral disease is no longer tenable. Psychoses of typical manic-depressive and schizophrenic kinds and psychogenic reactions can arise or recur in old age (Roth 1955), and follow-up studies (Kay 1962; Post 1962) have not shown that there is an excessive incidence of brain syndromes later or of deaths from cerebral disease; the average expectation of life, allowing for suicide, is not much below normal. Figure 1 shows the crude death rate in patients aged 60 or over with chronic brain syndromes and with functional disorders, admitted to the Stockholm mental hospital. Nearly all the patients were followed until their death. Compared with functional disorders, and also with the general population, brain syndromes have a very high mortality. In the chronic forms expectation of life is on the average reduced by at least half, and the certified causes of death are mostly those rather vague conditions given in the case of very aged or debilitated persons ("senility," "bronchopneumonia," "myocardial failure"), which suggest that vitality has reached a

TABLE 1

	Acute or Subacute Brain Syndromes (Acute Confusional or Delirious States)	Chronic Brain Syndromes (Dementia)
1. Duration	Weeks or rarely months	Years, less often months
2. Onset	Acute	Insidious
3. Memory	Impairment of retention and recall of recent events. Remote memory may be preserved.	Memory of recent events impaired. Remote memory partially or markedly impaired.
4. Variability	Fluctuations in level of consciousness over short periods from lucidity to clouding.	No discernible fluctuations in consciousness but variation in degree of restlessness, excitability, coherence of talk.
5. Perceptual disturbances	Visual and/or auditory hallucinations of disturbing, terrifying kind.	Hallucinations may be disturbing, but often ill-defined, fleeting or absent.
6. Orientation	Disoriented with positive misidentification of environment and people. Phenomena of confabulation, double orientation, etc.	Disoriented, but responses to questions more likely to be negative, declining knowledge, or giving grossly inaccurate but unembroidered replies.
7. General intellectual function	If accessible, power of reasoning, abstraction, etc. may be found well preserved.	General intellectual ability markedly impaired.
8. Delusions	Persecuting, fearful quality. Variable but with some consistency and cohesion.	Ill-sustained and inconsistent ideas of theft or interference.
9. Affect	Fearful, apprehensive, perplexed. Variability marked.	Fatuous, apathetic, or euphoric, sometimes depressive coloring in early stages; less variable, especially in advanced stages.
10. Etiology	Acute extracerebral disease (cardiac or hepatic failure, respiratory or urinary infections), or recent limited acute cerebral lesion, or intoxications.	Extensive, chronic, progressive cerebral disease.

very low ebb, with failure of the vegetative centers. Acute syndromes arising in previously normal people show a characteristic pattern of outcome: early death due to the specific cause, or else, in most cases, restitution to normal mental function.

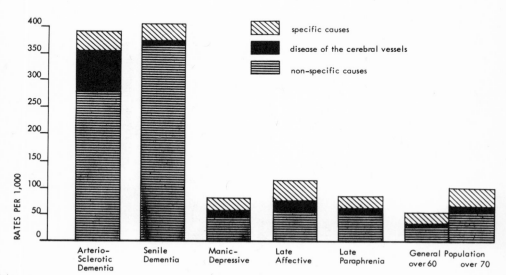

Figure 1. Crude mortality rates per 1,000 years of life in certain clinical groups admitted to a psychiatric hospital, and in the general population (Sweden 1931-1940). From Kay 1962. Reprinted with permission of the publisher, Acta Psychiatrica Scandinavica, *Risskov, Denmark.*

Neuropathological studies also indicate that the common chronic mental syndromes are due to structural damage to the brain, while the so-called functional disorders show as a rule age-related changes only (Corsellis 1962; Blessed, Tomlinson, and Roth 1968). When brain syndromes have been carefully distinguished from functional syndromes and from acute confusional states clinically, highly significant correlations between the diagnosis and the degree of change in the brain have been demonstrated. In the chronic syndromes, the changes are usually widespread and severe; in the brains of previously normal patients dying of systemic diseases, with or without an acute brain syndrome, and also in those of patients who have recently suffered from nonorganic mental disorders, changes may be absent or, if they exist as they usually do after the age of 70, they are nearly always mild (Roth 1971). Naturally, this distinction is not absolute and there is an area of overlap. But these findings give grounds for confidence in the validity of clinical and epidemiological findings in respect to chronic brain syndromes.

Epidemiology

Statistics from mental hospitals in developed countries show that over one third of the places are occupied by elderly patients. Unfortunately, for our purpose, residency rates are contaminated by the inclusion of many patients, such as aging schizophrenics, who have merely grown old in hospitals. First admission rates specific for age are more revealing (Figure 2). These show that the proportion of admissions due to brain

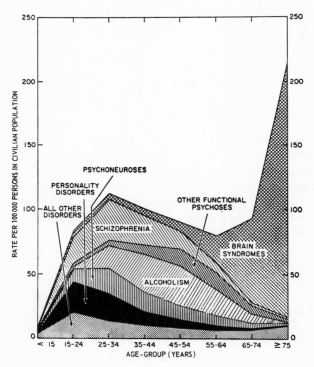

Figure 2. Rates for first admission to state and county mental hospitals in the United States in 1965 and specific for age and mental disorder (no previous admission to any inpatient psychiatric facility). From Kramer 1969.

syndromes remains rather constant in the age groups between 20 and 50 at about 5 percent and then increases very rapidly. In the age group 65 to 74, about 75 percent of first admissions to state and county mental hospitals in the United States are due to brain syndromes, and at ages over 75, about 90 percent (Kramer 1969). In Britain the trend is similar, though it is only after the age of 75 that brain syndromes predominate over all other disorders. At younger ages brain syndromes are associated with a large number of miscellaneous conditions, including cerebral trauma, tumor, and embolism; poisoning from alcohol, drugs, or carbon monoxide; infections causing meningitis, encephalitis, or neurosyphilis; and hereditary diseases such as Huntington's chorea. Any of these and many others can occur in the elderly, but the increase in age-specific admission rates is mainly due to two new groups of diseases, the vascular and senile (and presenile) degenerations. Acute brain syndromes associated with systemic diseases also contribute to the increase in the admission rates since they are much more common in old people.

Unfortunately there is little exact information about the epidemiology of acute brain syndromes. Those occurring in previously normal people form 10 to 25 percent of all brain syndromes among elderly patients in psychiatric admission wards and observation wards (Kay and Roth 1955; Simon and Tallery 1965). Males outnumber females perhaps by about two to one (Kay and Roth 1955). A physical disturbance is nearly always demonstrable, but the part played by aging of the brain itself is not clear. The importance of these acute syndromes is underlined by a recent recommendation of a World Health Organization scientific group (1970) that a rubric for "acute confusional states" should be added to the International Classification of Diseases to assist in exploring their epidemiology and associations with various diseases.

Large numbers of old people with brain syndromes, both acute and chronic, are found in acute medical and surgical wards, in annexes of general hospitals ("chronic sick" wards), and in residential and nursing homes. Probably at any one time 1 to 2 percent of the aged population are in these institutions suffering from brain syndromes. Admission to an institution, however, is often the result of a combination of medical, psychiatric, and also social factors (such as poverty or childlessness), and gives little indication of the prevalence of the disorder in the community at large.

Epidemiological surveys which include people living outside hospitals are confronted by the usual problems of case definition and identification. The earlier surveys, summarized by Lin (1953), are now of historical interest only. Relatively low rates for mental illness in the aged were reported, presumably because only the most severe cases were identified; families often do not consider their aging members as ill unless they become hallucinated, excited, or violent. Later studies, aimed exclusively at old people and often based on personal interviews with them, have generally yielded much higher estimates of mental illness (Table 2). The wide measure of agreement between different authors, often working in vastly different cultures, suggests that age-related biological phenomena are being recorded. Such differences as exist may be due to differences in criteria or method. For example, in the Swedish study of Åkesson (1969), who used an inquiry method, the prevalence of chronic brain syndromes was only 0.95 percent, but only those people who were "constantly disoriented" were counted. In another study from Sweden (Hagnell 1966 and 1970), 441 people aged 60 years or over were revisited after an interval of ten years, and during this time 40 (9.1 percent) of them were found to have developed a "senile psychosis" causing severe disability. The average annual incidence for mild, moderate, and severe disability from senile psychosis was estimated to be 2 percent, after making an adjustment for those who had died. When the

TABLE 2

Prevalence of Chronic Brain Syndromes at Ages 65 and Over

Author	Country	N(65+)	Dementia % 'Severe'	'Mild'	Remarks
Gruenberg	U.S.A.	1,592	6.8	–	'Psychosis of aging'
Primrose	Scotland	222	4.5	–	
Nielsen	Denmark	978	3.1	15.1	
Kay et al. (1964)	England	505	5.6	5.7	
Parsons	England	228	4.4	10.0	Domiciliary
Kaneko	Japan	531	7.2	–	
Hagnell	Sweden	441*	9.1	7.0	'Senile psychosis' 10-year period
Akesson	Sweden	4,198	1.0	–	'Constantly disoriented'
Kay et al. (1970)	England	758	6.2	2.6	Domiciliary

*60 and over

reported rates are based on personal interviews (Kay, Beamish, and Roth 1964; Kay et al. 1970; Kaneko 1967; Parsons 1965), they are usually a little higher than those based on second-hand information (Nielsen 1962). It may be concluded that in many parts of the world between 4 and 6 percent of the population aged 65 and over suffer from a definite chronic brain syndrome and that a further proportion have milder degrees of impairment. After making allowance for age, the sexes are generally found to be about equally affected.

All statistics and surveys agree that brain syndromes become increasingly more frequent beyond the age of 60 or 65 (Table 3). There seems to be a sharp rise after 80 when as many as one fifth of the population may be affected.

TABLE 3

Prevalence of Chronic Brain Syndromes by Age

	Japan	England	Denmark
N	696	758	994
65 –	2.3[1]	2.3	0
70 –	5.9	3.9	1.9
80 –	19.8	22.0	13.2
All ages	4.4	6.2	3.1

[1] 60–69

Arteriosclerotic and Senile Dementia

So far all types of chronic brain syndrome have been combined, because this is the way authors have usually reported their data. Very roughly, about one sixth of the cases may be due to other conditions, the remainder to senile and vascular disease. To separate these in surveys one has to rely on simple criteria. We have diagnosed arteriosclerotic dementia when, in the presence of a brain syndrome, the patient had a history of a cerebral accident or of fits with hypertensive disease, or when there was a neurological syndrome, and other causes of focal damage were excluded. Thus senile dementia comes to be diagnosed mainly by exclusion of cases with definite evidence of focal damage. This procedure seems to work quite well in practice, though the occurrence of fits, parietal lobe features or, perhaps, a confusional episode during the course of an illness with insidious onset and hitherto gradual progression may cause some uncertainty. We have tended to call such cases senile rather than arteriosclerotic. On this basis dementias of senile and vascular type seem to be, roughly, equally prevalent.

On the whole, fairly good correlation has been found between the clinical and neuropathological diagnoses (Roth 1971), provided that quantitative rather than "all or none" measures of cerebral change are used and that the degree of vascular change is assessed by the amount of brain tissue destroyed, and not merely by the degree of arteriosclerosis of the vessels. In about 20 percent of demented patients examined at autopsy, however, both types of change have been observed to be present in more than mild degrees. In these cases the senile and vascular changes appear to have potentiated each other in causing the dementia. Clearly, the occurrence of a vascular syndrome does not exclude the presence of senile change, and the co-existence of senile change should be suspected when, for example, a single stroke is followed by progressive mental deterioration.

The sex ratio is of interest (Table 4). Our survey findings indicate that arteriosclerotic dementia is somewhat more common in males and senile dementia in females,

TABLE 4

Prevalence of Main Types of Chronic Brain Syndrome by Sex and Age —
Newcastle upon Tyne

	Senile		Vascular		Other		Total	
	M	F	M	F	M	F	M	F
65 —	0.5	1.0	2.0	0.3	1.0	1.0	3.5	2.4
75 —	4.4	9.3	6.7	2.3	1.1	1.2	12.2	12.7
All ages	1.7	4.1	3.4	1.1	1.0	1.1	6.2	6.2

which accords with clinical impressions; but the question is not settled. The epidemiology of vascular dementia is bound up with the epidemiology of stroke and hypertension. Roughly about 50 percent of patients with arteriosclerotic dementia are hypertensive, and hypertensive disease takes a more malignant course in males. However, a systematic study of death certificates did not reveal a sex difference in the prevalence of cerebrovascular disease (Larsson 1967). The findings reported by Larsson, with the sexes combined, may be seen in Table 5. In another study the incidence of strokes over a ten-year period in previously unaffected old people was found to be similar in males and females (Hagnell 1970), though males tended to be affected at an earlier age. Males also became mentally disturbed after strokes more often than females, an observation that may help to reconcile some of the conflicting evidence.

As regards senile dementia, the life-time risks of contracting this disease have been calculated to be 1.8 percent for males and 2.1 percent for females (Larsson, Sjögren, and Jacobson 1963). The difference was considered to be too small to place much confidence in.

Mild Dementia

Surveys among old people living outside hospital have usually disclosed that a proportion of them, ranging from under 5 to 15 percent (Table 2) appear to be mentally dull, apathetic, forgetful, or out of touch with events, but are able to carry on their routine lives and to fulfill a limited social role. The presence of a brain syndrome may be suspected but the criteria are not fully met and a category of "mild dementia" is created. The existence of such a category raises many questions. How often do definite brain syndromes develop later? How long does the prodromal stage last, and how does it differ from normal senescent change? Do psychological tests help to detect the syndrome before it has become clinically obvious?

It is well known that performance on some psychological tests tends to fall progressively at higher ages. For example, in a large-scale investigation of age and function a battery of tests was given to normal people who were very carefully selected so as to represent all age groups from 20 up to 80 years (Heron and Chown 1967). In the age group 70 to 79, in males, the best score on the Progressive Matrices test was equal to the average score of the 20- to 29-year-old group, and many of the older people achieved very poor scores indeed on this and on certain other tests (Figure 3). One gets the impression, looking at these data, that at still higher ages some people would not have been able to score at all, and it is tempting to try to relate these and similar findings to the mild dementias reported during survey work, and also to the generally mild neuropathological changes that occur with aging in nondemented old people (Tomlinson, Blessed, and Roth 1968).

Now, according to the "aging theory" of senile dementia, this is merely an exaggerated form of the usual decline that occurs as people grow old, presumably due, at least in part, to a gradual accumulation of senile changes (Roth 1971). A clinically recognizable brain syndrome arises, according to this theory, when a certain threshold or critical degree of change has been reached, resulting in disorganization of everyday behavior. The "mildly demented" and perhaps, too, the poor test performers, could be thought of as approaching but not having quite reached this threshold. The different ages at which people are affected would be due to a number of factors, including perhaps genetic ones, but everyone would be affected if they lived long enough.

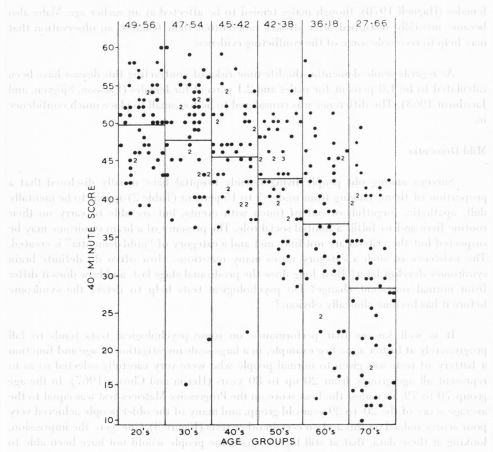

Figure 3. Scores on Progressive Matrices (men). Distribution of 40-minute scores with means indicated by horizontal lines and by figures at top of each column. From Heron and Chown 1967.

This model is attractive because it brings together observations from different disciplines. There is, however, an absence of studies that correlate psychological, clinical, and pathological data. The main alternative theory was put forward by the Swedish authors on the basis of their massive work on senile dementia (Larsson, Sjögren, and Jacobson 1963) (Table 5). In a family study, these authors found that the first-degree relatives of patients with senile dementia were about four times as liable to the disease as corresponding age groups in the general population, and they concluded that a single dominant gene would best account for their findings. Such a gene might be present in 12 percent of the population, and its "penetrance" would increase with age, so that by the

TABLE 5

Aggregate Morbidity Risks in Senile Dementia
and in Cerebrovascular Disease (Percentages)

| Up to age | Senile dementia | | Cerebrovascular disease |
	Gen. pop.	First-degree relatives	Gen. pop.
50	—	—	0.4
60	—	0.2	1.2
70	0.4	2.0	4.4
75	1.2	5.7	8.8
80	2.5	11.3	16.0
85	3.8	16.9	29.0
90	5.2	23.0	45.0

(1) Aggregate morbidity risks (percentages) for senile dementia in general population
and in first degree relatives (Larsson, Sjögren, and Jacobson 1963).
(2) Aggregate morbidity risks for cerebrovascular disease based on study of death
certificates (Larsson 1967).

age of 90 about 40 percent of the carriers would be affected. An important piece of evidence in support of this theory, and against the "aging theory," was the apparent absence of relatives showing intermediate states between "normal senility" and senile dementia (and, it may be added, of relatives with Alzheimer's disease).

If the major-gene theory is correct, only those who carry the gene will become demented, and the prodromal stage may elude detection with ordinary tests. If the aging theory is correct, chronic brain syndromes should be found to develop only after a period of gradual deterioration differing only in degree from the changes of normal senescence.

Actually there is very little information about the later history of these so-called "mild dementias." Among psychiatric patients suffering from functional disorders, in whom the presence of "mild organic mental symptoms" suggested the possibility of an early brain syndrome, and in residents of old people's homes who showed "senescent forgetfulness" (in contrast to "malignant amnesia"), there appeared to be no special risk of the development of a brain syndrome in the usual sense (Kay 1962; Kral 1962). In a follow-up in Newcastle of 711 people aged 65 years and over, 30 were found to have developed chronic brain syndromes two to four years after the initial interviews, an annual average incidence of 1.4 percent (Bergmann et al. 1971). Of these 30, an early brain syndrome had been originally suspected in only 6. Thus, in only 0.5 percent of the whole sample was a brain syndrome successfully predicted. These findings seem to suggest that some other factor in addition to age-related change is necessary to create the conditions for a fully developed chronic brain syndrome.

Some Implications of Epidemiological Studies and Future Research

Organic brain disease in the aged is closely related to the biological processes that result in aging and death, which is one cogent reason for concentrating effort in this area. Senile dementia itself, however, forms only a part of the totality of brain syndromes, and impaired mental function, either temporary or permanent, may be caused by a large number of conditions, some of which are capable of being prevented or treated by the application of methods that are already available. Extension of knowledge in this area offers the greatest hope of prolonging useful life. However, as duration of life increases, so the risk of senile dementia also increases. Its relationship to normal senescence here becomes of crucial importance. Psychological testing of representative samples of old people seems to show that if the average duration of life were prolonged for a few more years, there would be a great number of mentally enfeebled old people, but their intellectual functions would be affected unevenly, and they might not be seriously disabled in everyday life. It is possible that there are two forms of "senile dementia," one a mild, gradual process closely related to aging, the other qualitatively distinct from normal aging, more severe in its effect, and akin to Alzheimer's presenile dementia. It is of interest that the "gnostic disorders," traditionally held to distinguish Alzheimer's disease from senile dementia, have recently been reported to be present in many, though not all, patients with senile dementia (Lauter and Meyer 1968).

From the social point of view, any upward change in total population or its age structure will increase the number of people with malfunctioning brains. On this basis alone, it was estimated in Sweden that the number of places in mental hospitals would need to be more than doubled between 1960 and 1980 (Larsson, Sjögren, and Jacobson 1963). If in addition there was a greater demand for places, such as might occur with changing social attitudes and rising standards and expectations, then the number would be nearly trebled. What are the alternatives to mental hospital care? Already the greater part of the burden is falling on the families. Various schemes are being tried or have been proposed. Conditions, however, differ greatly from one region to another, and operational research on a regional basis and on a limited scale is needed to assess the merits and demerits of different programs. It will be desirable, for example, to assess the feasibility of programs in terms of cost and manpower, and the effects they have on the quality of life of the old people themselves and on their families (Grad and Sainsbury 1965).

References

Åkesson, H.O. 1969. A population study of senile and arteriosclerotic psychoses. *Human Heredity* 19:546.

Bergmann, K.; Kay, D.W.K.; McKechnie, A.A.; Foster, E.; and Roth, M. 1971. Paper read at International Congress of Psychiatry, Mexico City.

Blessed, G.; Tomlinson, B.E.; and Roth, M. 1968. The association between quantitative measures of dementia and of senile change in the cerebral grey matter of elderly subjects. *Brit. J. Psychiat.* 114:797.

Corsellis, J.A.N. 1962. *Mental Illness and the Aging Brain.* Maudsley Monograph No. 9. London: Oxford University Press.

Grad, J.; and Sainsbury, P. 1965. An evaluation of the effects of caring for the aged at home. In *Psychiatric Disorders in the Aged.* Manchester: Geigy (U.K.) Ltd., p. 225.

Gruenberg, E.M. 1961. *A Mental Health Survey of Older People.* New York: Utica.

Hagnell, O. 1966. *A Prospective Study of the Incidence of Mental Disorder.* New York: Humanities Press.

Hagnell, O. 1970. Disease expectancy and incidence of mental illness among the aged. *Acta Psychiat. Scand.* suppl. 219, p. 83.

Heron, A., and Chown, S. 1967. *Age and Function.* London: Churchill.

Kaneko, A. et al. 1967. Kosei no Shihyo (Health Statistics) 14:25.

Kay, D.W.K. 1962. Outcome and cause of death in mental disorders of the aged: a long-term follow-up of functional and organic psychoses. *Acta Psychiat. Scand.* 38:249.

Kay, D.W.K.; Beamish, P.; and Roth, M. 1964. Old age mental disorders in Newcastle upon Tyne. Part I: A study of prevalence. *Brit. J. Psychiat.* 110:146.

Kay, D.W.K.; Bergmann, K.; Foster, E.M.; McKechnie, A.A.; and Roth, M. 1970. Mental illness and hospital usage in the elderly: a random sample followed up. *Compr. Psychiat.* 11:26.

Kay, D.W.K., and Roth, M. 1955. Physical accompaniments of mental disorder in old age. *Lancet* 2:740.

Kral, V.A. 1962. Senescent forgetfullness: benign and malignant. *Canad. Med. Assoc. J.* 86:257.

Kramer, M. 1969. *Application of Mental Health Statistics.* Geneva:World Health Organization.

Larsson, T. 1967. Mortality from cerebrovascular disease. In *Stroke.* A. Engel and T. Larsson (eds.). Stockholm: Nordiska Bokhandelns Förlag, p. 15.

Larsson, T.; Sjögren, T.; and Jacobson, G. 1963. Senile dementia. *Acta Psychiat. Scand.* 39, suppl. 167.

Lauter, H., and Meyer, J.E. 1968. Clinical and nosological concepts of senile dementia. In *Senile Dementia.* C. Müller and L. Ciompi (eds.). Stuttgart: Huber.

Lin, T. 1953. Mental disorder in Chinese and other countries. *Psychiatry* 16:313.

Nielsen, J. 1962. Geronto-psychiatric period-prevalence investigation in a geographically delimited population. *Acta Psychiat. Scand.* 38:307.

Parsons, P.L. 1965. Mental health of Swansea's old folk. *J. Prev. Soc. Med.* 19:43.

Post, F. 1962. *The Significance of Affective Symptoms in Old Age.* London: Oxford University Press.

Primrose, E.J.R. 1962. *Psychological Illness: A Community Study.* London: Tavistock Publications.

Roth, M. 1955. The natural history of mental disorders arising in the senium. *J. Ment. Sci.* 101:281.

Roth, M. 1971. Classification and aetiology in mental disorders of old age: some recent developments. In *Recent Developments in Psychogeriatrics.* D.W.K. Kay and A. Walk (eds.). Ashford (U.K.): Headley Bros.

Simon, A., and Malamud, N. 1965. Comparison of clinical and neuropathological findings in geriatric mental illness. In *Psychiatric Disorders in the Aged.* Manchester: Geigy Ltd., p. 322.

Simon, A., and Tallery, J.E. 1965. The role of physical illness in geriatric mental disorders. In *Psychiatric Disorders in the Aged.* Manchester: Geigy Ltd., p. 154.

Tomlinson, B.E.; Blessed, G.; and Roth, M. 1968. Observations on the brains of non-demented old people. *J. Neurol. Sci.* 7:331.

World Health Organization Report of Scientific Group on Psychogeriatrics. October 1970.

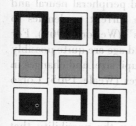

Aspects of Neuropsychological Assessment in Patients with Cerebral Disease

Arthur L. Benton, Ph.D., and
Maurice W. Van Allen, M.D.

Neurosensory Center and Departments of
Neurology and Psychology, University of Iowa
Iowa City, Iowa

Psychological impairment associated with brain disease takes a great variety of forms, depending primarily on the locus, extent, and nature of the cerebral lesion and secondarily on premorbid characteristics of the patient, e.g., his intellectual level, his personality, and his hemispheric cerebral organization as reflected (imperfectly) in his lateral preference. Assessment of the various forms of behavioral impairment associated with brain disease has a two-fold interest. First, it is of theoretical interest in that it provides data from which inferences about cerebral organization and the functional properties of the different areas of the brain can be made. Secondly, from a practical standpoint, it provides a relatively accurate and unbiased estimate of various aspects of a patient's behavioral capacity which can aid diagnosis and management in various ways, e.g., in making a judgment about the presence of cerebral disease in the doubtful case, in furnishing a baseline against which future changes in status can be measured, as a guide in rehabilitation, and in providing evidence for focal cerebral disease in the form of specific cognitive, perceptual, or psychomotor deficits.

Neuropsychological assessment is based on evaluation of performance. In making such an assessment, it is necessary to keep constantly in mind that a patient's behavior has multiple determinants and that his cerebral status in the neurological sense is only one of those determinants. Level of energy and motivation, attitudinal factors and physical disabilities other than brain disease can alter performance to a significant degree.

NOTE: The investigative work described in this presentation was supported by Research Grant NS-00616 and Program-Project Grant NS-03354 from the National Institute of Neurological Diseases and Stroke.

The necessity to take account of other factors in making inferences about cerebral status from behavioral evaluation perhaps applies with particular force when older patients are the subject of study. Decline in performance in older subjects as compared either to younger age groups or to their own performances in the past is, of course, the rule. It is natural to try to relate this performance decline to what is generally known about CNS changes with age, e.g., loss of cerebral neurons, senile plaque formation, vascular disease, and fiber degeneration in the spinal cord. But the significance of such factors as alterations in attitude and mood, physical debility, and peripheral neural and non-neural changes as determinants cannot be ignored, despite current tendencies to minimize their importance as compared to "central mechanisms" (Welford 1969). For example, impairments in various aspects of visual perception in old age are quite possibly conditioned by decreased transparency of the lens, reduction in pupil size, and changes in the vitreous humor as well as by CNS (including retinal) changes (Weale 1965; Corso 1971).

The purpose of these introductory remarks is not to deny the possibility that behavior can be related to cerebral status in either normative or clinical studies of older people but simply to point out that other variables of a physical or psychological and social character have to be taken into account if broad inferences about the nature of this relationship are to be drawn.

Different approaches can be taken to the neuropsychological assessment of a patient or a normal person, depending upon one's interests and goals. The outline we will sketch reflects two interrelated but distinctive interests. The first is of a clinical nature, namely, to provide information that will help the clinical neurologist in his evaluation and management of a patient. The second aim is of a theoretical nature, namely, to provide information bearing on some persisting problems in the area of brain-behavior relationships, e.g., the association between locus of lesion and pattern of test performance, the distinctive functional properties of different cerebral areas, the cerebral organization of abilities as reflected in certain syndromes, and the nature of aphasic, agnosic, and apraxic disorders.

From a clinical standpoint, perhaps the first purpose of neuropsychological assessment is to obtain an estimate of overall mental efficiency in order to determine whether dementia (i.e., a general decline in mental ability) is present and, if so, its severity. Admittedly the concept of "dementia" is not very satisfactory from a theoretical point of view since it is rather vague and loosely defined. But the concept is of tremendous pragmatic importance to the physician who needs predictive measures of a patient's capacity to cope with the demands of everyday life. From an operational standpoint, dementia is assessed by comparing the score made by a patient on a battery of mental tests with the score that would be expected on the basis of his background, the difference between the scores being interpreted as a measure of decline from his premorbid intellectual level. Any reasonably comprehensive series of tests such as the Wechsler Adult Intelligence Scale (WAIS), the Halstead battery, or less elaborate test batteries can be used for this purpose.

In addition to providing an index of general mental impairment which has obvious clinical significance, the total score derived from a test battery is probably the best single index of the presence of cerebral disease in the doubtful case (Chapman and Wolff 1959; Reitan 1959; Fogel 1964; Vega and Parsons 1967). Nor is such a general measure devoid of neurological significance, despite the criticisms which have been levelled against it. In their monumental study, Chapman and Wolff (1959) found that the Wechsler-Bellevue IQ and the Halstead Impairment Index correlated to a highly significant degree with estimated amount of tissue loss in patients with excised neoplasms. Similarly, Blessed, Tomlinson, and Roth (1968) have reported a substantial correlation (r=.59) between the score on a brief test battery assessing orientation, memory, and concentration and the number of senile plaques found in the brains of older patients.

The Chapman-Wolff study found that Wechsler Performance Scale IQ correlated much more closely with size of lesion than did the Verbal Scale IQ. This result parallels the established finding that scores on the WAIS Performance Scale subtests decline with age much more precipitously than do scores on the Verbal Scale subtests (Birren et al. 1963).

On the negative side, one has to concede that current test batteries have certain limitations despite this evidence of a highly significant association between the global indexes and the presence or severity of cerebral disease. First, a lack of concordance between the test measures (which may indicate only slight impairment) and the quite obvious behavioral incompetence of a patient may be observed. In this respect, it is of interest that Blessed, Tomlinson, and Roth found that a direct assessment of behavioral competence obtained from relatives of the patients and covering such areas as changes in habits, personality, and the performance of everyday activities correlated even more closely (r=.77) with the estimated amount of loss of cortical neurons than did the scores on their test battery. Second, the test batteries apparently are not sufficiently sensitive to detect minor degrees of general mental impairment which probably underlie the complaints of loss of memory and inability to concentrate by some patients. The fault here may be of a technical nature. No great amount of thought has gone into the assembling of tests in current diagnostic batteries, and it is probable that a more judicious selection of tests to form a battery expressly designed to detect the presence and severity of mental impairment associated with cerebral disease would lead to more impressive results.

In any case, both for clinical purposes and for theoretical reasons, considerable emphasis is placed today on eliciting evidence of specific behavioral defects of various types, e.g., impairment of retention and memory, visuoperceptive and visuoconstructive disabilities, disturbances in skilled motor performance, and decline in language functions. The philosophy behind this approach is that the evaluation of specific performances will yield distinctive information about brain function not provided by any single index derived from a test battery (Spreen and Benton 1965). Some of these tests will be described and the results of their application discussed with reference to both brain disease and old age. Because of their current interest, we shall focus on procedures designed to assess the functions of the right hemisphere, i.e., the so-called "minor" hemisphere. At the same time, it is hardly necessary to review once again such functions as reaction time (King 1965; Talland 1965; Botwinick 1970) or learning and memory (Botwinick and Birren 1963; Inglis 1965; Botwinick 1970) which have been covered so thoroughly in the recent literature.

As is well known, during the past 20 years considerable evidence has been accumulated to indicate that certain types of cognitive performances are mediated primarily by the right hemisphere. This evidence is derived for the most part from observation of selective performance deficits in patients with unilateral cerebral disease with some support from the study of normal subjects and patients with section of the corpus callosum. An adequate definition of these performances in terms of underlying abilities still eludes us, but one prominent feature is that they often deal with the spatial aspects of nonsymbolic material.

It is in the field of visuoperceptive and visuoconstructive performances that most of the work concerned with the functional properties of the right hemisphere has been done. Some representative studies will be described to show what the outcome of this work has been.

Meier and French (1965) studied visual discrimination in patients who had undergone resection of either the right or the left temporal lobe for psychomotor seizures, the two groups having been equated for age and WAIS IQ. The task assessed the ability to discriminate between circular patterns on the basis of either rotational or structural cues (Figure 1). The patients with right hemisphere lesions were clearly inferior to those with left hemisphere excisions, their mean error score being 46 per cent higher, and the intergroup difference in mean error score being significant at the .01 level.

In a similar study, Warrington and James (1967a) investigated the perception of incomplete figures by patients with right or left hemisphere disease. The tasks they

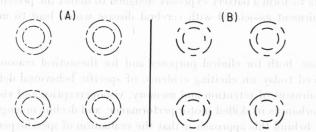

Figure 1. Sample items in visual discrimination task of Meier and French (1965).

employed are shown in Figure 2. The patients with left hemisphere damage performed on a normal level and this was true of subgroups defined in terms of temporal lobe involvement, parietal lobe involvement, or the presence of aphasia. In contrast, the patients with right hemisphere damage performed significantly worse than either the controls or the left hemisphere group on two of the three perceptual tasks. Further analysis showed that the subgroup of patients with right parietal disease were particularly severely impaired.

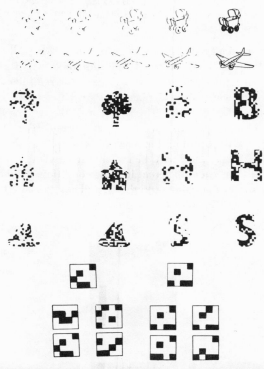

Figure 2. Sample items in incomplete figures task and retention task of Warrington and James (1967).

Another type of performance which has received considerable attention in studies of patients with unilateral lesions is facial recognition. The reason for the choice of this rather unusual task as an investigative procedure is that occasionally a patient is encountered whose primary complaint is that he is unable to recognize familiar people by inspection of their faces. This curious disability (called "facial agnosia" or "prosopagnosia") is generally associated with the presence of disease of the right hemisphere (Hécaen and Angelergues 1962), and it can appear within a context of unimpaired intelligence, vision, and language functions. Since facial agnosia is rather rare, at least in relatively pure form, clinical researchers have turned to study of the capacity of patients with cerebral disease to discriminate representations of unfamiliar faces, the assumption being that this procedure would probe the same cognitive and perceptual abilities as those involved in the recognition of faces of familiar persons (De Renzi and Spinnler 1966; Warrington and James 1967b; De Renzi, Faglioni, and Spinnler 1968; Benton and Van Allen 1968; Tzavaras, Hécaen, and Le Bras 1970; Yin 1970). As it happens, the assumption has been shown to be unfounded in the sense that the disabilities underlying facial agnosia and impairment in performance on the visuoperceptual task of discriminating unfamiliar faces are, or at least may be, dissociable (Benton and Van Allen 1972). On the other hand, the experimental task has proved to be of interest in its own right since it has been found to be associated with disease of the right hemisphere.

For example, in our own study (Benton and Van Allen 1968), defective performance (defined as a score below the distribution of scores of a large control group) was shown by 40 percent of the patients with lesions of the right hemisphere as compared to 4.5 percent of patients with left hemisphere disease. Three types of task constitute the test, as illustrated in Figures 3, 4, and 5. The first part of the test requires the matching of identical front-view photographs of faces. In the second part, the subject matches front-view photographs with three-quarters view photographs of the same person on the multiple choice display. In the third part, he matches front-view photographs of the same person that have been taken under different lighting conditions. Thus, while the first part of the test presents a simple matching task, the second and third parts require the patient to perceive identity within diverse configurations.

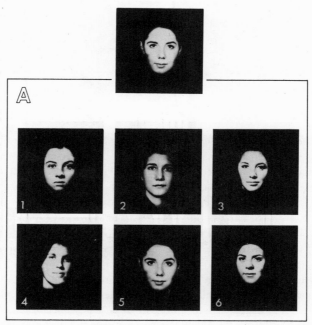

Figure 3. Item in Part A of facial recognition test of Benton and Van Allen (1968).

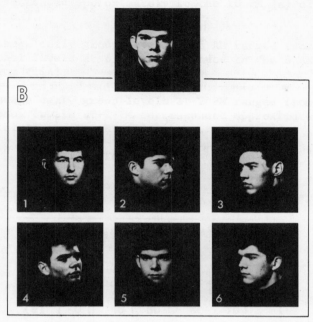

Figure 4. Item in Part B of facial recognition test of Benton and Van Allen (1968).

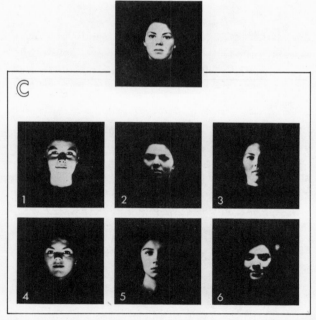

Figure 5. Item in Part C of facial recognition test of Benton and Van Allen (1968).

We have only limited observations on the performances of older normal subjects, but such data as we have indicate that there is a progressive decline in performance level with age. Table 1 presents some statistics for three age groups. The decrease in mean score is obvious, but the indications are that this is not associated with an increase in variability. The lower mean scores of the older age groups seem to be determined more by a failure to attain very superior levels of performance than by the increased occurrence of grossly inferior performances. These indications need to be validated by the collection of considerably more data on the performances of older subjects. If they should be confirmed, it is possible that this task, performance on which is related to the function of the right hemisphere, can be utilized to advantage in the clinical evaluation of older persons.

TABLE 1

Scores on Facial Recognition Test of

Control Patients in Different Age Groups

| | Age Range | | |
	16-55 Yrs. (N = 107)	56-65 Yrs. (N = 34)	66-70 Yrs. (N = 7)
Mean	45.6	42.1	40.4
s	4.2	3.5	3.8
Range	35-54	34-51	34-48

Another type of task that has figured prominently in studies of patients with unilateral brain disease with special reference to the functions of the right hemisphere involves various types of constructional performance, e.g., block building, and mosaic assembling as in block designs tests. The copying of designs is also counted among these constructional tasks.

A substantial amount of evidence derived from study of patients with unilateral cerebral disease indicates that impairment in visuoconstructive performances (so-called "constructional apraxia") tends to be both more frequent and more severe in patients with lesions of the right hemisphere than in those with lesions of the left hemisphere (Benton 1967; Warrington 1969). At the same time, impairment in left hemisphere damaged patients is by no means rare, and indeed those with receptive language disorder are likely to show as much constructional deficit as an unselected group of patients with right hemisphere disease (Dee, Benton, and Van Allen 1970).

Table 2 presents the findings of a recent study of the performances of patients with right or left hemisphere disease on four constructional tasks (Benton 1967). Defining impairment as a performance level exceeded by 95 percent of control patients, it appears that the strength of the tendency toward a higher frequency of deficit in patients with right hemisphere disease is related to the specific task employed. While defective performance on design copying and block construction is more than twice as frequent in the right hemisphere group as in the left hemisphere group, the differences between the groups for stick constructions and block designs are minimal. These relationships change somewhat when only quite severe impairment is considered; here a trend toward a higher frequency of defect in the right hemisphere group is seen for all the tests.

TABLE 2

Visuoconstructive Deficits in Patients with Lesions
of the Right and Left Hemispheres[1]

Test	Deficit[2]			Severe deficit[3]		
	Right %	Left %	R/L Ratio	Right %	Left %	R/L Ratio
Design copying	29	14	2.1	14.5	5	2.9
3-Dimensional block construction	54	23	2.3	23	9	2.6
Stick construction	34	26	1.3	14	7	2.0
Block designs	34	30	1.1	20	14	1.4

[1]Benton (1967).

[2]Performance level below that of 95 to 100 percent of control patients (N=100).

[3]Performance level below that of 100 percent of control patients.

We have only partial information on the relationship between these task performances and age in control patients since 65 years is the upper limit of the age range of patients in our studies. In one study of 100 control patients ranging in age from 18 to 65 years, block designs showed a small but significant negative association (r=−.25) with age. The other constructional tests failed to show significant relationships to age.

The latter, however, present very easy tasks for normal subjects and this circumstance precludes disclosing any possible relationships with age for these types of performance. For example, 90 of 100 control patients made perfect performances on the three-dimensional block construction task. On the other hand, a modification of the task in which the patient was required to make his constructions on the basis of photographs instead of actual block models resulted in a systematically lower level of performance with only 35 percent making perfect scores. With this task a lower performance on the part of patients within the 50 to 60 years age range as compared to that of younger patients was evident (Benton and Ellis 1970).

These visuoperceptive and visuoconstructive performances, impairment in which appears to have a quantitatively close relationship to disease of the right hemisphere, represent only a sample of wide range of performances that show a similar relationship, e.g., visual depth perception (Carmon and Bechtoldt 1969; Benton and Hécaen 1970), certain forms of auditory discrimination (Milner 1962; Kimura 1963; Vignolo 1969), some tactile-proprioceptive functions (Carmon and Benton 1969; Carmon 1970; Fontenot and Benton 1971), and certain motor performances (Berlin 1955; Fisher 1956; Joynt, Benton, and Fogel 1962). There is no assurance that their application to the study of normal and pathological aging would yield information not already provided by more conventional test methods. However, the circumstances that these procedures have been investigated in relation to a number of neurological and psychological variables in younger subjects suggests that the undertaking might be fruitful.

References

Benton, A.L. 1967. Constructional apraxia and the minor hemisphere. *Conf. in Neurol.* 29:1.

Benton, A.L., and Ellis, E.E. 1970. Test de praxie tri-dimensionnelle: observations normatives concernant la performance au test lorsque les stimuli sont des photographies de constructions-modèles. *Rev. Psychol. Appl.* 20:255.

Benton, A.L., and Hécaen, H. 1970. Stereoscopic vision in patients with unilateral cerebral disease. *Neurology* 20:1084.

Benton, A.L., and Van Allen, M.W. 1968. Impairment in facial recognition in patients with cerebral disease. *Cortex* 4:344.

Benton, A.L., and Van Allen, M.W. 1972. Prosopagnosia and facial discrimination. *J. Neurol. Sci.* 12 in press.

Berlin, L. 1955. Compulsive eye opening and associated phenomena. *Arch. Neurol. Psychiat.* 73:597.

Blessed, G.; Tomlinson, B.E.; and Roth, M. 1968. The association between quantitative measures of dementia and of senile change in the cerebral grey matter of elderly subjects. *Brit. J. Psychiat.* 114:797.

Birren, J.E.; Botwinick, J.; Weiss, A.D.; and Morrison, D.F. 1963. Interrelations of mental and perceptual tests given to healthy elderly men. In *Human Aging*. J.E. Birren et al. (eds.). Washington D.C.: Public Health Service Publication No. 986, p. 111.

Botwinick, J. 1970. Geropsychology. *Ann. Rev. Psychol.* 21:239.

Botwinick, J. and Birren, J.E. 1963. Mental abilities and psychomotor responses in healthy aged men. In *Human Aging*. J.E. Birren et al. (eds.). Washington D.C.: Public Health Service Publication No. 986, p. 97.

Carmon, A. 1970. Impaired utilization of kinesthetic feedback in right hemisphere lesions. *Neurology* 20:1033.

Carmon, A., and Bechtoldt, H.P. 1969. Dominance of the right cerebral hemisphere for stereopsis. *Neuropsychologia* 7:29.

Carmon, A., and Benton, A.L. 1969. Tactile perception of direction and number in patients with unilateral cerebral disease. *Neurology* 19:525.

Chapman, L.F., and Wolff, G.H. 1959. The cerebral hemispheres and the highest integrative function of man. *Arch. Neurol.* 1:357.

Corso, J.F. 1971. Sensory processes and age effects in normal adults. *J. Geront.* 26:90.

Dee, H.L.; Benton, A.L.; and Van Allen, M.W. 1970. Apraxia in relation to hemispheric locus of lesion and aphasia. *Trans. Amer. Neurol. Assoc.* 95:147.

De Renzi, E.; Faglioni, P.; and Spinnler, H. 1968. The performance of patients with unilateral brain damage on face recognition tasks. *Cortex* 4:17.

De Renzi, E., and Spinnler, H. 1966. Facial recognition in brain-damaged patients. *Neurology* 16:145.

Fisher, M. 1956. Left hemiplegia and motor impersistence. *J. Nerv. Ment. Dis.* 123:201.

Fogel, M.L. 1964. The intelligence quotient as an index of brain damage. *Amer. J. Orthopsychiat.* 34:555.

Fontenot, D.J., and Benton, A.L. 1971. Tactile perception of direction in relation to hemispheric locus of lesion. *Neuropsychologia* 9:83.

Hécaen, H., and Angelergues, E. 1962. Agnosia for faces (prosopagnosia). *Arch. Neurol.* 7:92.

Inglis, J. 1965. Immediate memory, age and brain function. In *Behavior, Aging and the Nervous System.* A.T. Welford and J.E. Birren (eds.). Springfield: Thomas, p. 88.

Joynt, R.J.; Benton, A.L.; and Fogel, M.L. 1962. Behavioral and pathological correlates of motor impersistence. *Neurology* 12:876.

Kimura, D. 1963. Right temporal lobe damage. *Arch. Neurol.* 8:264.

King, H.E. 1965. Psychomotor changes with age, psychopathology and brain damage. In *Behavior, Aging and the Nervous System.* A.T. Welford and J.E. Birren (eds.). Springfield: Thomas, p. 476.

Meier, M.J., and French, L.A. 1965. Lateralized deficits in complex visual discrimination and bilateral transfer of reminiscence following unilateral temporal lobectomy. *Neuropsychologia* 3:261.

Milner, B. 1962. Laterality effects in audition. In *Interhemispheric Relations and Cerebral Dominance.* V.B. Mountcastle (ed.). Baltimore: Johns Hopkins Press, p. 177.

Reitan, R.M. 1959. The comparative effects of brain damage on the Halstead Impairment Index and the Wechsler-Bellevue Scale. *J. Clin. Psychol.* 15:281.

Spreen, O., and Benton, A.L. 1965. Comparative studies of some psychological tests for cerebral damage. *J. Nerv. Ment. Dis.* 140:323.

Talland, G.A. 1965. Initiation of response, and reaction time in aging, and with brain damage. In *Behavior, Aging and the Nervous System.* A.T. Welford and J.E. Birren (eds.). Springfield: Thomas, p. 526.

Tzavaras, A.; Hecaen, H.; and Le Bras, H. 1970. Le problème de la spécificité du déficit de la reconnaissance du visage humain lors des lésions hémisphériques unilatérales. *Neuropsychologia* 8:403.

Vega, A., and Parsons, O.A. 1976. Cross-validation of the Halstead-Reitan tests for brain damage. *J. Consult. Psychol.* 31:619.

Vignolo, L.A. 1969. Auditory agnosia: a review and report of recent evidence. In *Contributions to Clinical Neuropsychology.* A.L. Benton (ed.). Chicago: Aldine, p. 172.

Warrington, E.K. 1969. Constructional apraxia. In *Handbook of Clinical Neurology, Volume 4.* P.J. Vinken and G.W. Bruyn (eds.). Amsterdam: North-Holland, p. 67.

Warrington, E.K., and James, M. 1967a. Disorders of visual perception in patients with localized cerebral lesions. *Neuropsychologia* 5:253.

Warrington, E.K., and James, M. 1967b. An experimental investigation of facial recognition in patients with unilateral cerebral lesions. *Cortex* 3:317.

Weale, R.A. 1965. On the eye. In *Behavior, Aging and the Nervous System.* A.T. Welford and J.E. Birren (eds.). Springfield: Thomas, p. 307.

Welford, A.T. 1969. Age and skill: motor, intellectual and social. In *Decision Making and Age.* A.T. Welford and J.E. Birren (eds.). Basel: Karger, p. 1.

Yin, R.K. 1970. Face recognition by brain-injured patients: a dissociable ability? *Neuropsychologia* 8:395.

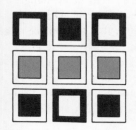

Neurochemistry of Aging

Thaddeus Samorajski, Ph.D.

Laboratory of Neurochemistry
Cleveland Psychiatric Institute, Cleveland, Ohio

J. Mark Ordy, Ph.D.

Department of Psychology,
Northern Illinois University, DeKalb, Illinois

Stimulated in part by rapid and parallel advances in biochemistry and neurobiology, the field of neurochemistry has been characterized by a remarkable expansion in the past decade. Despite this rapid advance, however, research on the neurochemistry of aging in man and other primates has been sparse and inconclusive. This paucity of research can be attributed in part to the long life span of man and the primates and in part to the broad, diversified, and exploratory focus on such biological mechanisms of aging as the extracellular components collagen and elastin, the search for age changes in particular cell types, tissue, or organs as a whole, and more recently the neuromolecular emphasis on age differences in a variety of intracellular organelles.

In contrast to the broader and diversified biological approach, the new field of neurochemistry exemplifies, by virtue of its subject matter, a more specific emphasis on one particular organ, i.e., the nervous system and its time-dependent neurochemical changes that may take place with advancing age. Although there may be some advantages for research in this selective emphasis on one particular organ, there are also subtle and unique disadvantages since the nervous system plays a critical role in the chemistry of the total organism. Also, the central nervous system is frequently sensitive to and affected by many metabolic disorders and hormonal imbalances that have an origin in other organs. These disorders and imbalances can have significant effects on the brain in aging but have only negligible effects on other organs of the body at younger age levels. Consequently, the unique integrating role of the nervous system may make it more difficult to identify, segregate, and interpret the time-dependent neurochemical changes that may occur with advancing age. This complexity provides one of the greater challenges for neurochemistry, but any progress can yield significant benefits to the individual and society.

Aging processes are important factors in a wide variety of diseases affecting the

41

nervous system. Some of the diseases are known to result from a genetically determined change in the level of an enzyme. In other cases, chemical changes in the brain appear to be secondary to a genetically determined defect in some specific area of metabolism, or they may arise from conditions not directly related to gene mutation, such as metabolic imbalance, vascular degeneration, and death of cells. Differentiation of primary defects from secondary changes presents numerous problems to the investigator since changes in pathologic states are frequently the result of an interaction between genetic background, environmental agents, and aging processes. In addition, there are many chemical changes that are known to occur in various neurological disorders that may interact with such normal ongoing morphological changes as the constant loss of neurons that takes place as part of the aging process. From the clinical standpoint, biochemical analysis of brain tissue may serve to provide an additional means of differentiating a disease from other related conditions or provide confirmation of a diagnosis. Progress in preventing and treating some of the disorders in which the nervous system is affected depends in part on understanding the nature of aging processes and the causative roles they play in disease.

Since the neurochemistry of aging is a relatively new branch of gerontology, it is still possible to sketch the major contemporary problems and highlights of some present controversies. The general aims of this review are to focus on those major current issues that may determine the direction and rate of future research rather than discuss in detail any one particular problem in the neurochemistry of aging. The subjects covered include: (1) age differences in the chemical composition of human brain, (2) species differences in the neurochemistry of aging, (3) chemical changes in subcellular components in aging brain, (4) research methods for manipulating age differences in the brain, and (5) theoretical considerations of neuronal aging.

Age Differences in the Chemical Composition of Human Brain

As in all new branches of science, certain issues and techniques available to investigators often become crucial determinants of the direction and rate of progress. For example, one of the current problems in the neurochemistry of aging is the assumption that aging in the brain is a consequence of some molecular changes occurring throughout the brain. Many biochemists have looked and continue to look for physical and chemical alterations at various age levels which would be deleterious to the brain. Another important consideration is the fact some changes may prove to be so characteristic that they may serve to differentiate stages of aging. It has been observed, however, that in many instances age-related changes did not occur or were confounded by the presence of chronic progressive organic brain disease. If we consider the chemical biomorphosis of human brain, we find that many lipid constituents such as neutral fats, cerebrosides, phosphatides, and total sterols, total nitrogen, and phosphorus content are unaltered or only slightly decrease with age (Figure 1). Significant declines occur in sulfur content, brain weight, and in oxygen consumption during comparable periods of aging. The numbers for DNA content in dry substance and percentage of water in human brain are progressively higher with increasing age.

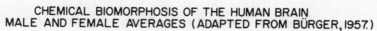

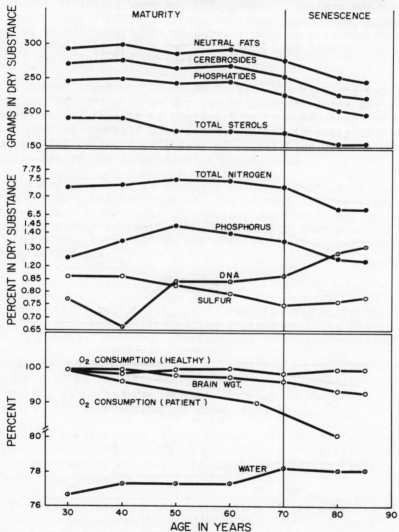

Figure 1. Changes in constituents, weight, and oxygen consumption of the human brain with aging.

For the purpose of comparison of brain composition at various age levels, a number of criteria have been considered in an effort to demarcate the period of senescence in the human being. Based on data for brain weight, water content, total solids and total lipids, it has been convenient to consider the age of 70 as the beginning of the period of senescence (Himwich and Himwich 1959). This is the time when important aging processes are believed to occur at the cellular level and chronic brain syndromes are common and very disabling in the elderly.

Species Differences in the Neurochemistry of Aging

Since most animal species have a shorter life span than man, most research in neurochemistry of aging has included lower species. Inbred and random-bred mice and rats are most commonly used. The chemical biomorphosis of some brain constituents of C57BL/10 mice is illustrated in Figure 2. Biochemical determinations reveal that RNA, serotonin, and total protein increase in the brain as a result of aging. DNA, water content, and brain weight remain unchanged, and acetylcholinesterase activity and norepinephrine content decrease significantly by 24 months of age. From comparative studies of man and lower species, it has become evident that significant species differences exist. For example, average brain wet weight in the human decreases from a mean value of 1320

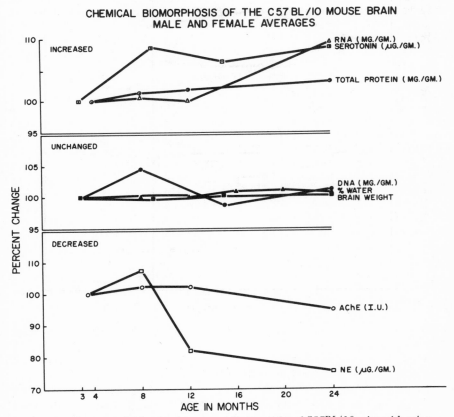

Figure 2. Changes in brain constituents and brain weight of C57BL/10 mice with aging.

grams at 21 years of age to 1225 grams by 70 years, a difference of approximately 7 percent. At the same time, there is a significant increase in water and DNA content (Himwich 1959; Himwich and Himwich 1959). In the mouse brain, mean wet weight, percentage of water, and DNA content change only slightly with increasing age (Figure 2).

Regional differences in the percentage of water content in human and mouse brain are graphically illustrated in Figure 3. The comparisons indicate that water content increases in the human and decreases in the mouse in corresponding regions with advancing age. Since the brain weight of man and some of its chemical constituents decline with advancing age while many of the same chemical constituents and brain weight of most lower animal species remain unchanged or increase, comparisons and generalizations from lower species to man require considerable caution. Unfortunately,

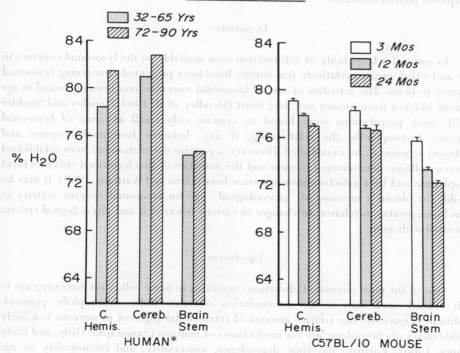

Figure 3. Changes in water content in the cerebral hemisphere, cerebellum, and brain stem of human and mouse brain at different age levels. The values increase with age for human brain and decrease for mouse brain.

very few biochemical data are available on the effects of aging in the brain of other species. Consequently, the selection of appropriate animal species that would permit generalizations from animal studies to man is an issue of considerable current importance in the neurochemistry of aging.

Chemical Changes in Subcellular Components in Aging Brain

Based on microscopic study of the nervous system, it has been often reported that the neuron density in various brain regions declines with age. The greatest decrease in the neuronal population is reported to occur in the cerebral cortex (Bondareff 1959). In some regions of the human brain more than 20 percent of the neurons may be lost by the seventh decade of life (Brody 1955). In addition to the numerical decrease in neurons in various areas of the brain, changes in various subcellular organelles and related constituents may also be associated with senescence. These are: (a) lysosomes, (b) lipofuscin and related inclusion bodies, (c) the cell nucleus, (d) endoplasmic reticulum (microsomes), (e) mitochondria, (f) membranes, (g) nerve endings, (h) the Golgi complex, and finally, (i) various extracellular components such as glial cells, blood vessels, and amorphous ground substance.

Lysosomes

In spite of a large body of information now available on the lysosomal enzymes in liver and other organs, relatively few studies have been presented concerning lysosomal enzymes in brain. The activities of several lysosomal enzymes have been measured in age pigment isolated from human and beef heart (Hendley et al. 1963; Hendley and Strehler 1965). Such preparations were found to contain only small amounts of lysosomal enzymes. Consequently the relationship, if any, between lysosomal enzymes and lipofuscin remains to be extablished. However, a positive correlation has been established between collagen denaturation tension and the activities of two lysosomal enzymes (acid phosphatase and beta galactosidase) in mouse liver (Elens and Wattiaux 1969). It may be possible to obtain a measure of "physiological" age for lysosomal enzyme activity in brain homogenates in relation to changes in various behavioral and physiological criteria associated with aging.

Lipofuscin

One of the most consistent alterations occurring in nerve cells with increasing age in both animals and man is the accumulation of intracellular sudanophilic pigment, lipofuscin (Figure 4). The relative amount of intracellular pigment in neurons is a fairly reliable index of chronologic age for most classes of neurons (Samorajski, Ordy, and Rady Reimer 1968). Further, the time dependence, universality, and intrinsicality of age pigments have lead several investigators to suggest that they may be a major factor in the aging process (Strehler 1960; Björkerud 1964). Chemical analysis reveals that lipofuscin contains predominantly phospholipids (Strehler and Mildvan 1962), some of which may

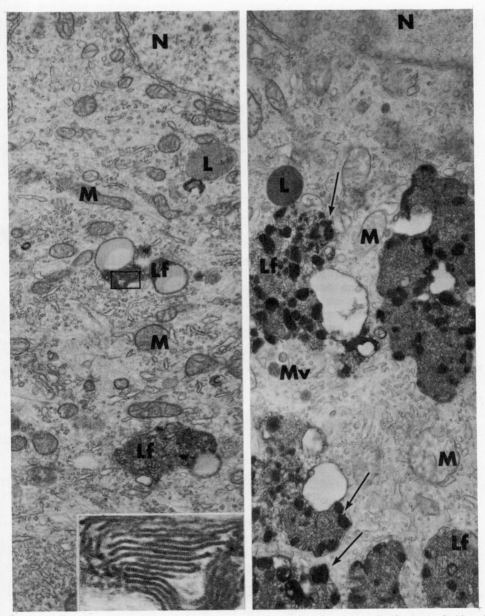

Figure 4. Electron micrographs of dorsal root ganglion cells of a 4-month-old mouse (left) and 30-month-old mouse (right). Vacuolated lipofuscin pigment bodies (Lf) with curved bands (insert) and lysosomes (L) are visible in both cells. Also identified are nuclei (N), mitochondria (M), and a multivesicular body (Mv). The lipofuscin bodies of the 30-month-old mouse contain many dense crystal-like particles (arrows). Some of the mitochondria of the older animal appear larger and more irregular in outline than the mitochondria in the ganglion cell of the young animal. X 16,200 and X 17,000, left to right; insert X 120,000. (From Samorajski, Ordy, and Rady Reimer 1968)

represent the only abnormal form of lipid present in brain of aging subjects. The functional significance of lipofuscin pigment accumulation in neonatal tissue has not been clarified, however, and attempts to isolate pigment from human brain have not been entirely successful. During the isolation procedure the physical properties of brain pigment appear to be altered as evidenced by a change in their fluorescent characteristics. Consequently, it must be assumed that alterations in the chemical composition of the pigment may be occurring as well. In addition, the extreme anatomical heterogeneity and the chemical and functional complexity of the nervous system make it very difficult to interpret any biochemical information obtained by isolation procedures at a level higher than a small group of neurons.

There are many reports of an increase in lipofuscin or ceroid in the brain in several diseases (Zeman and Alpert 1963; Donahue, Zeman, and Watanabe 1966; Kristensson and Sourander 1966; Pallis, Duckett, and Pearse 1967) and in various experimental conditions (Sulkin and Srivanij 1960; Miyagishi, Takahata, and Iizuka 1967; Földi, Zoltán, and Györi 1970; Várkonyi et al. 1970). The identification of lipofuscin pigment in the nervous system of experimental animals and man poses several important problems. First, it is not known whether the accumulation of lipofuscin and the other types of inclusion bodies found in the nervous system represents a distinct metabolic process with a specific chemical characterization, or whether similar metabolic processes are involved in each case, differentiated only by the age at which they become evident. Second, it is not known whether the accumulation of lipofuscin pigment is associated with any functional impairment and cell destruction. Finally, it has not been established whether the process of pigment accumulation can be altered by chemical interaction. Germane to the future course of research is whether accumulation of pigment is related in any way to life span and the overall aging process.

Recently, Alzheimer plaques and central cores have been the subject of intensive study by several groups of investigators. During the past year Nikaido and associates (1971) succeeded in isolating small quantities of Alzheimer plaques and cores for biochemical analysis. Progress thus far indicates that there may be a slight increase in mucopolysaccharides, glycogen, and hexuronic acids in Alzheimer cortex. Presumably these changes reflect an abnormal collection of neurofibrillar and microtubular structures referable both to neurons and glia (Terry 1963; Terry, Gonatas, and Weiss 1964; Wiśniewski, Terry, and Hirano 1970). A reduction in other moieties was considered to be consistent with the observation of some cell loss in the cortex. Numerous other inclusion bodies are found in a variety of diseases that affect the brain. Some of these bodies may be confused with lipofuscin since they also contain phospholipids and may be similar histochemically and ultrastructurally.

Studies of irradiation effects on cell metabolism, particularly in relation to free-radical damage and lipofuscin accumulation in nerve cells, may offer some interesting possibilities for research on aging at the cellular and subcellular level. For example, it is not known whether pigment formation can be accelerated by irradiation and, if so, whether an accelerated accumulation would correlate with an early cell loss. There is now good evidence to suggest that age pigments are derived from lysosomes and that the ratio of lysosomes to age pigments differs with age. Efforts to control the lysosome-to-lipofuscin ratio by chemical intervention remains as an interesting problem for future investigations.

Nuclei

There are several lines of evidence suggesting various types of nuclear abnormalities associated with neuronal aging. It is now widely accepted that the information necessary for the control of cell function is encoded in the deoxyribonucleic acid of the chromosomes, and that control is mediated by the DNA-directed synthesis of ribonucleic acid (Wulff et al. 1967). Thus, the genetic material DNA is an obvious candidate for the primary chemical alteration in aging since each molecule has a unique biological function. Recently, evidence has been presented suggesting that with aging the nuclear DNA in certain brain cells may accumulate damage such as simple strand breaks (Price, Modak, and Makinodan 1971). *In vitro* experiments have shown that the chemical and physical properties of DNA are significantly altered by radiation. The similarity between radiation damage and aging has been noted by many investigators. However, at the present time, there is little or no evidence for a quantitative change in nuclear DNA with age. Studies on brain tissue as well as on the liver reveal that DNA per nucleus, nuclear volume, and the number of nuclei per unit area of tissue remains essentially constant with age (Andrew 1964). The overall biosynthetic capacity of the nerve cell, however, seems to diminish with age (MacKinnon, Simpson, and MacLennan 1969). It has been shown that maximum incorporation into both DNA and RNA after injection of ^{32}P-phosphate is reached later in old rats than in young animals, and the labeled phosphorus is lost at a slower rate in older animals (Nikitin and Shereshevskaia 1961 [cited by Oeriu 1964]). These changes in turnover in the brain of the rat may be related to a decrease in protein content, a relative accumulation of RNA, and an increase in the protease-to-ribonuclease ratio during the period of senescence (Umaña and Brekke 1969).

Endoplasmic Reticulum (Ribosomes)

Age-dependent changes in endoplasmic reticulum (microsomes) are strongly suggested by the decrease in the amount of Nissl substance observed in nerve cells of older animals and humans. Nissl bodies are granular RNA-containing concentrations of endoplasmic reticulum (Palay and Palade 1955).

Recent investigations of rat brain RNA have shown that the amount of transfer RNA as well as ribosomal RNA may be dependent on both age and learning. It has also been found that the proportion of polysomes bound to the rough endoplasmic reticulum decreases with increasing age, and that the amino acid acceptor capacities of transfer RNA may be age-dependent. From these and other findings, it has been postulated that the biochemical disturbances that develop in the brain with aging may be a consequence of a reduction in the "precision, predictability, and functional efficiency" of molecular systems involved in the synthesis of RNA and of protein (Gordon 1971). It is tempting, also, to speculate that protein synthesis in the endoplasmic reticulum may be under the influence of hormone action and novel incoming stimuli, some of which may be originating from degenerating cells in other regions of the body. The elucidation of the exact interrelationships between these molecules and nucleic acid and protein synthesis in the neuron presents some of the most challenging problems for future research.

Mitochondria

Very little is known about the fate of mitochondria in brain cells during aging. Measurements of mitochondrial concentration on electron micrographs of hepatic cells of human (Tauchi and Sato 1968) and pyramidal tract fibers of mouse brain (Samorajski, Friede, and Ordy 1971) revealed that the number of mitochondria in a given area of cytoplasm may decrease with age. Besides the decrease in mitochondrial concentration with age, an increase in size and number of bizarrely shaped mitochondria may be noticed in the liver. Similar differences in morphology may be expected in some cell types of the nervous system.

The chemical components of mitochondria in vertebrates show little difference in relation to organ, species, and age. Changes in the rate of turnover of certain mitochondrial constituents, however, may be an important characteristic of senescence in post-mitotic cells. Following injection of labeled precursor, the radioactivity of mitochondrial DNA and lipids per unit weight of protein in brain is found to be decreased with age (Huemer et al. 1971). Changes in oxidative phosphorylation and respiratory control of brain mitochondria have not been accurately evaluated, chiefly because of technical difficulties in isolating mitochondria from different cell types in the nervous system.

Membranes

Lipid accounts for more than one-half of the dry weight of the adult human central nervous system and is a major constituent of the plasma membrane. However, lipid metabolism in the brain is not well understood at any age level, and for the most part the enzymes involved in lipid synthesis and degradation have not been characterized adequately. During the past decade it has been supposed that gray-matter lipids had an appreciable turnover while the myelin lipids were quite inert except during early myelination. Recent studies in several laboratories including our own have shown that these suppositions are probably not true. Figure 5 illustrates the progressive increase in myelin content in mouse and rat brain, even with advanced age.

The ethanolamine phosphoglycerides (glyceryl-3-phosphorylethanolamine—GPE) are major components of membrane isolated from the brain. Table 1 illustrates the turnover rates of diacyl GPE and alk-l-enyl GPE in membrane fractions of mitochondria,

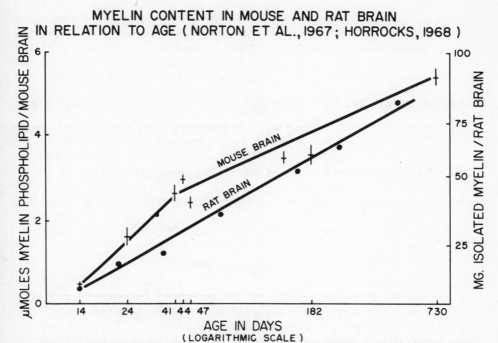

Figure 5. Changes in myelin content in mouse and rat brain in relation to age (14 to 730 days).

TABLE 1

The Half-Life of Ethanolamine Phosphoglycerides Isolated from Mouse Brain
Subcellular Fractions after Intracerebral Injections of ^{14}C-Ethanolamine
(Horrocks 1969 and unpublished)

	Age at Injection		
	40 Days	150 Days	730 Days
Mitochondria			
diacyl GPE*	–	1.9	7.9
alk-l-enyl acyl GPE	–	2.4	6.3
Microsomes			
diacyl GPE	1.3	1.9	6.9
alk-l-enyl acyl GPE	1.3	2.4	10.3
Myelin			
diacyl GPE	1.7	3.0	10.3
alk-l-enyl acyl GPE	1.6	3.2	20.3
Cytosol (supernatant)			
total radioactivity	–	1.1	5.8

*GPE = glyceryl-3-phosphorylethanolamine

microsomes, myelin, and supernatant after intracerebral injections of ^{14}C-ethanolamine into mice of three different ages. Note that the half-life of each of these fractions increases markedly as a function of age and that the myelin lipids turn over at a slower rate than other brain membranes. It is probable also that the plasma membrane of the cell wall, as well as nuclear membranes, are in a continual process of turnover (Strehler 1962).

The fatty acid composition of ethanolamine phosphoglycerides in myelin isolated from human brain at three different age levels is shown in Figure 6. There is a relative increase with age in the proportion of the monoenoic fatty acids (18:1 and 20:1) and a decrease in the polyunsaturated fatty acids (20:4, 22:4, and 22:6). Age-related changes have been observed also in other phospholipids of total human brain homogenate (Rouser and Yamamoto 1969).

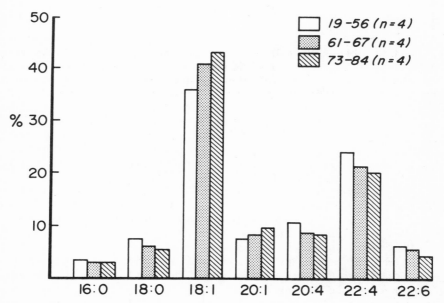

Figure 6. Changes in fatty acid composition of ethanolamine phosphoglycerides in human myelin in relation to age.

Only a small amount of research is now being conducted on the basic biochemistry of neuronal membranes during the aging process. Also, isolation procedures now in use are inadequate for isolating pure membrane fractions and they provide variable results. Caution in interpreting the available data is indicated in view of the multiplicity of cell types present in the brain and the unknown influence of species, diet, and disease on the lipids of subcellular particles. Determination of the lipid compositions and protein structure of the plasma membranes of the nervous system in relation to age is a difficult and challenging task.

Nerve Endings

A number of investigators have attempted to relate biochemical changes in the synapse to age and various types and periods of stress. Changes in acetylcholinesterase activity, norepinephrine content, and serotonin concentration in brain homogenates of mice have been associated with increasing age (Samorajski, Rolsten, and Ordy 1971). Electric-shock stress for 15 days altered norepinephrine and acetylcholinesterase concentrations to a variable degree dependent on the age of the animals. However, the exact relationship between neurotransmitter substances and synaptic ultrastructure remains problematic because of the regional differences in the synthesis and storage of these substances in the nervous system and peripheral tissues. Nerve-ending particles isolated from brain may prove to be useful subcellular systems for biochemical investigations of age changes at the synaptic level (Sun and Samorajski 1970).

The Golgi Complex

Age-associated changes in the Golgi apparatus of mouse sympathetic ganglia have been described (Gatenby 1953). There is little agreement with what these morphologic changes are, however, and still less about their significance in aging. It would appear from several lines of evidence that the Golgi complex may be only part of an extensive membrane system extending throughout the cell (Palade 1955). Isolated Golgi components have high specific concentrations of acid phosphatase and phospholipid and seem to be involved in storage and possibly modification of some substances (Dalton 1961). The Golgi complex has been isolated in pure enough form to allow the beginning of age-related biochemical analyses.

Extracellular Components

The interaction between nerve cells and their extracellular environment represents a relatively unexplored facet of gerontology. Changes in glial cells, blood vessels, and constituents of the extracellular ground substance which may accompany aging would probably have a profound effect on the function of individual cells or groups of cells in the nervous system. The presence of a small number of labeled cells in the brain of aged mice after injection of ^{3}H-thymidine indicates that some cells do proliferate, even at an advanced age (Dalton, Hommes, and Leblond 1968). The successful isolation of glia from the central nervous system for biochemical and morphologic analysis may provide a suitable means of studying these elements at various age levels (Norton and Poduslo 1970; Raine, Poduslo, and Norton 1971).

The physical and chemical characteristics of arteriocapillary fibrosis commonly observed in the brain of aged individuals and after irradiation have not been adequately defined and the role of blood vessels in the aging processes of the brain remains largely unknown. The application of biochemical techniques to extracellular substance has not been sufficiently thorough to permit any generalization concerning the role of this material in aging.

Research Methods for Manipulating Age Differences in the Brain

Behaviorally, a decrease in the speed of response is one of the most characteristic changes in the aging organism (Birren 1959 and 1965). It has been shown in both human beings and animals that reaction time becomes progressively slower with aging. However, various diets (McCay 1952; Silberberg and Silberberg 1955; Harman 1971), exercise (Retzlaff and Fontaine 1965), and stress (Ordy et al. 1967) may alter the rate and possibly delay the onset of physiological aging. It is evident from previous work that age and/or stress can have some important consequences on chemical constituents of the brain (Smookler and Buckley 1969), ultrastructural characteristics of selected fiber tracts of the brain and certain peripheral nerves (Samorajski and Friede 1968; Friede and Samorajski 1968; Samorajski, Friede, and Ordy 1971), and neuroendocrine organs (Geller, Yuwiler, and Zolman 1965; Dixit and Buckley 1969). Rats exposed to forced exercise have a higher average life span than "no-exercise" animals and the sciatic nerves of the exercised group at 900 days of age had an average conduction velocity of 45M/sec; whereas the no-exercise group had an average of only 20M/sec (Retzlaff and Fontaine 1965). Underfeeding of rats may also produce a significant increase in life span (McCay 1952). From these and other findings, it may be hypothesized that a variety of "extrinsic" environmental factors exert a beneficial effect on the aging organism. On the other hand, a number of mutant mice having disorders in the development and function of the nervous system have shortened life spans. Some of these mice (Jimpy mutant) manifest a sudden onset of neurological symptoms and rarely survive after 30 days of age. Others (Ataxic mutant) reveal a progressive neurologic motor disability early in life but apparently live a normal life span. Human progeria has been characterized pathologically as premature aging (Reichel and Garcia-Bunuel 1970).

Several lines of evidence indicate that radiation can simulate some of the more specific effects of aging in cells as well as accelerate many of the more obvious structural and functional changes observed normally with aging (Ordy et al. 1967; Samorajski et al. 1970; Ordy et al. 1971). After whole-body irradiation at levels ranging from 500 to 2,500 rads, most experimental subjects die within 80 to 500 hours as a result of a bone marrow syndrome. At ranges between 2,500 rads and 12,500 rads the animals die in about 80 hours from gastrointestinal causes. Both conditions result from damage to proliferating cell systems. At doses above 12,500 rads, death occurs within a few minutes to 80 hours depending on dose, as a result of neuronal damage secondary to edema (CNS syndrome). Partial-body irradiation also induces life shortening. We have recently found that focal irradiation of the brain at dose levels below 25,000 rads decreases survival time from causes unknown in approximate relation to the dose of irradiation administered (Figure 7). Surprisingly, a plot of the mortality rate of the irradiated mice versus survival time revealed a logarithmic relation (Ordy et al. 1971). The mortality rate of humans and infrahuman species is a logarithmic function of age also (Strehler 1962).

From all of the foregoing studies, it is apparent that a variety of experimental means is available for manipulating and relating age changes in such unique functions as learning and memory to certain electrophysiological, biochemical, and cellular changes in various regions of the brain.

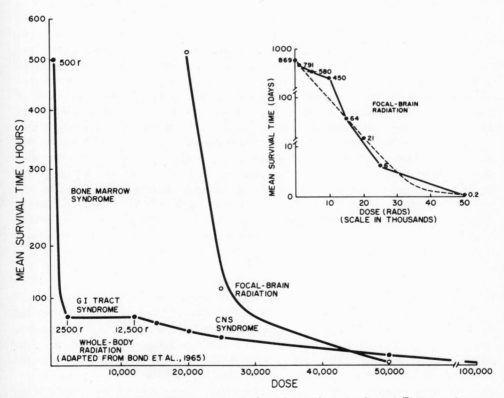

Figure 7. Mean survival time following whole-body and focal brain irradiation. The curve for mean survival after focal brain irradiation was drawn free-hand from a plot of data (upper right of figure) obtained in a study of changes in longevity of adult mice after exposure of the brain to cyclotron-accelerated focal deuteron beams (Ordy et al. 1971).

Theoretical Consideration of Neuronal Aging

Although varying considerably in detail, current biological theories of aging can be divided into two general and contrasting categories (Curtis 1963; Strehler 1966). According to probabilistic or stochastic theories, environmental factors including stress can influence mortality, longevity, and the rate of aging. A variety of evidence has been presented in support of these "wear-and-tear" theories of aging. In contrast to these theories, deterministic molecular and genetic theories have proposed that post-maturity aging is genetically programmed and similar to early maturation and growth. These post-maturity changes in the brain and other organs with age are presumed to result primarily from an accumulation of defects in DNA or in DNA-directed metabolic activity. Within each of these two broad categories, there are numerous other theories and mathematical models that have attempted to provide a coherent and integrated interpretation of aging.

Although aging has been tentatively defined in genetic-molecular theories primarily as an invariant or DNA-"programmed" biological transformation in cells with time, this has not excluded the possibility that environmental stressors or stimuli may interact with the so-called primary DNA-"programmed" biological processes of aging and modify the onset as well as the rate of aging. However, there is as yet insufficient experimental evidence to exclude various contending theoretical views concerning the interaction between genetically "programmed" and environmental factors involved in biological aging. Very few experimental studies have examined the specific interaction effects between genetically "programmed" and "environmental" influences in the biological rate of aging of the central nervous system and other regulatory mechanisms in relation to cell loss and age changes in behavior, mortality, and longevity. Recent behavioral and biochemical ontogenetic studies have demonstrated, however, that the developing central nervous system may undergo a variety of morphological, biochemical, and functional changes in response to even subtle environmental fluctuations or conditions (Krech, Rosenzweig, and Bennett 1966; Ring, Bosch, and Lo 1970). However, no similar observations have been reported on the role of environmental influences, stress, or disease in the subsequent biological aging of the central nervous system in relation to age changes in behavior, mortality and longevity.

Methodologically, one of the more urgent current needs is the development of appropriate experimental designs or models for obtaining and evaluating, either by cross-sectional or longitudinal designs, data on small but significant chemical changes that may occur in the brain under conditions of accelerated aging or during an extended period of the life history of a species with different variances at each age level. In summary, it seems clear that the future direction and rate of progress in the neurochemistry of aging will depend on: (1) defining "chemical senescence" of the brain within the entire ontogenetic sequence for man and lower animal species; (2) the simultaneous focus on whole brain, regional, and molecular chemical changes during aging; (3) the selection of higher animal species for study; and (4) the use of appropriate experimental designs for evaluating small but physiologically significant changes in the brain.

Summary

Since the neurochemistry of aging is one of the most recent areas of research in gerontology, the focus of research seems to be directed toward time-dependent age differences in molecular components of the brain in general accord with the contemporary emphasis on molecular mechanisms in the entire field of biology. It seems important to note, however, that even at this stage of neurochemical research the search for molecular age changes in the brain may not provide an exclusive or parsimonious explanation of biological aging. In contrast to the molecular search for aging, age changes may occur in the properties of different cell types, regions, or the brain as a whole that are more uniquely associated with aging. Brain size, for example, represents one of the most significant parameters of any organ of the mammalian body that shows a large range of variability independent of body size. Although no essential molecular differences in the brain among different species have been established, there is a significant correlation between brain size and life span in phylogeny.

Another unique feature of the brain as an organ or system is the progressive cell loss of post-mitotic neurons which are not replaced by cell division in the adult mammalian brain. There seems to be general agreement that the appearance of many behavioral and physiological manifestations of aging for the organism as a whole may also be associated with the progressive loss of neurons from the brain. Although most neurochemists are aware of the possible effects of the internal environment and disease processes in other organs and their effect on the brain in aging, recent studies with several animal species have suggested that the external environment may also exert an influence on the chemistry of the brain throughout the post-maturity period of the life span. In summary, although considerable reserve or redundancy seems to be a characteristic of the brain in common with other organs, the lack of cell replacement with advancing age and deleterious effects of the internal and external environment on the brain must all have serious implications or consequences for the progressive age changes in behavior, neurophysiology, and neurochemistry of the organism.

The chemical changes occurring in discrete areas of the brain in response to various disease processes are difficult to assess from the data available. The problems of the variation in samples from corresponding anatomical areas of diseased brain and differences between autopsy material as compared to biopsy samples add to the confusion created by the paucity of data available. We still do not know why certain diseases, virtually unknown in the young, manifest themselves in the aged. It might be expected that the study of chemical constituents of brain over the entire period of life would add to our knowledge of the critical changes associated with disease and senescence.

Acknowledgments

The authors are indebted to Dr. Howard J. Curtis, Dr. Reinhard L. Friede, Dr. C.P. Baker, Dr. Lloyd A. Horrocks, and their staffs for their kind cooperation in these studies. Assistance provided by Dr. Grace Sun, Miss Carolyn Rolsten, and Mrs. Nancy Terlop is gratefully acknowledged.

References

Andrew, W. 1964. Changes in the nucleus with advancing age of the organism. In *Advances in Gerontological Research*. B.L. Strehler (ed.). New York: Academic Press, vol. 1, p. 87.

Birren, J.E. 1959. Sensation, perception and modification of behavior in relation to the process of aging. In *The Process of Aging in the Nervous System*. J.E. Birren, H.A. Imus, and W.F. Windle (eds.). Springfield, Ill.: Charles C Thomas, p. 143.

Birren, J.E. 1965. Age changes in speed of behavior: Its central nature and physiological correlates. In *Behavior, Aging, and the Nervous System*. A.T. Welford and J.E. Birren (eds.). Springfield, Ill.: Charles C Thomas, p. 191.

Björkerud, S. 1964. Isolated lipofuscin granules: A survey of a new field. In *Advances in Gerontological Research*. B.L. Strehler (ed.). New York: Academic Press, vol. 1, p. 257.

Bond, V.P.; Fliedner, T.M.; and Archambeau, J.O. 1965. *Mammalian Radiation Lethality: A Disturbance in Cellular Kinetics*. New York: Academic Press, p. 276.

Bondareff, W. 1959. Morphology of the aging nervous system. In *Handbook of Aging and the Individual*. J.E. Birren (ed.). Chicago: The University of Chicago Press, p. 136.

Brody, H. 1955. Organization of the cerebral cortex. III. A study of aging in the human cerebral cortex. *J. Comp. Neurol.* 102:511.

Bürger, M. 1957. Die chemische Biomorphose des menschlichen Gehirns. Abhandlungen der Sachsischen Akademie der Wissenschaften zu Leipzig, *Mathematisch-naturwissenschaftliche Klasse* 45:1.

Curtis, H.J. 1963. Biological mechanisms underlying the aging process. *Science* 49:626.

Dalton, A.J. 1961. Golgi apparatus and secretion granules. In *The Cell: Biochemistry, Physiology, Morphology*. J. Brachet and A.E. Mirsky (eds.). New York: Academic Press, p. 603.

Dalton, M.M.; Hommes, O.R.; and Leblond, C.P. 1968. Correlation of glial proliferation with age in the mouse brain. *J. Comp. Neurol.* 134:397.

Dixit, B.N., and Buckley, J.P. 1969. Brain 5-hydroxytryptamine and anterior pituitary activation by stress. *Neuroendocrinology* 4:32.

Donahue, S.; Zeman, W.; and Watanabe, I. 1966. Electron microscopic observations in Batten's disease. Proceedings Third International Symposium on The Cerebral Sphingolipidoses. Reprinted from *Inborn Disorders of Sphingolipid Metabolism*. New York: Pergamon Press, p. 3.

Elens, A., and Wattiaux, R. 1969. Age-correlated changes in lysosomal enzyme activities: An index of ageing? *Exp. Geront.* 4:131.

Földi, M.; Zoltán, O. T.; and Györi, I. 1970. Über die Wirkung von Kavain und Magnesium-Orotat auf die funktionellen Störungen bei der experimentellen lymphogenen Enzephalopathie. I. Mitteilung. *Z. Geront.* 3:97.

Friede, R.L., and Samorajski, T. 1968. Myelin formation in the sciatic nerve of the rat. *J. Neuropath. Exp. Neurol.* 27:546.

Gatenby, J.B. 1953. The Golgi apparatus of the living sympathetic ganglion cells of the mouse, photographed by phase contrast microscopy. *J. Roy. Micr. Soc.* 73:61.

Geller, E.; Yuwiler, A.; and Zolman, J.F. 1965. Effects of environmental complexity on constituents of brain and liver. *J. Neurochem.* 12:949.

Gordon, P. 1971. Molecular approaches to the drug enhancement of deteriorated functioning in the aged. In *Advances in Gerontological Research*. B.L. Strehler (ed.). New York: Academic Press, vol. 3, p. 199.

Harman, D. 1971. Free radical theory of aging: Effect of the amount and degree of unsaturation of dietary fat on mortality rate. *J. Geront.* 26:451.

Hendley, D.D.; Mildvan, A.S.; Reporter, M.C.; and Strehler, B.L. 1963. The properties of isolated human cardiac age pigment. II. Chemical and enzymatic properties. *J. Geront.* 18:250.

Hendley, D.D., and Strehler, B.L. 1965. Enzymic activities of lipofuscin age pigments: Comparative histochemical and biochemical studies. *Biochim. Biophys. Acta* 99:406.

Himwich, H.E. 1959. Biochemistry of the nervous system in relation to the process of aging. In *The Process of Aging in the Nervous System.* J.E. Birren, H.A. Imus, and W.F. Windle (eds.). Springfield: Charles C Thomas, p. 101.

Himwich, W.A., and Himwich, H.E. 1959. Neurochemistry of Aging. In *Handbook of Aging and the Individual.* J.E. Birren (ed.). Chicago: The University of Chicago Press, p. 187.

Horrocks, L.A. 1968. Composition of mouse brain during development. *J. Neurochem.* 15:483.

Horrocks, L.A. 1969. Metabolism of ethanolamine phosphoglycerides of mouse brain myelin and microsomes. *J. Neurochem.* 16:13.

Horrocks, L.A. Content, composition and metabolism of mammalian and avian lipids that contain ether groups. In *The Ether Bond in Lipids.* F. Snyder (ed.). New York: Academic Press (in press).

Huemer, R.P.; Bickert, C.; Lee, K.D.; and Reeves, A.E. 1971. Mitochondrial studies in senescent mice. I. Turnover of brain mitochondrial lipids. *Exp. Geront.* 6:259.

Krech, D.; Rosenzweig, M.R.; and Bennett, E.L. 1966. Environmental impoverishment, social isolation and changes in brain chemistry and anatomy. *Physiol. Behav.* 1:99.

Kristensson, K., and Sourander, P. 1966. Occurrence of lipofuscin in inherited metabolic disorders affecting the nervous system. *J. Neurol. Neurosurg. Psychiat.* 29:113.

MacKinnon, P.C.B.; Simpson, R.A.; and MacLennan, C. 1969. *In vivo* and *in vitro* techniques used in the study of RNA synthesis in the brains of rats and mice at various ages from birth to senility. *J. Anat.* 104:351.

McCay, C.M. 1952. Chemical aspects of ageing and the effect of diet upon ageing. In *Cowdry's Problems of Ageing.* A.I. Lansing (ed.). Baltimore: Williams and Wilkins, p. 139.

Miyagishi, T.; Takahata, N.; and Iizuka, R. 1967. Electron microscopic studies on the lipo-pigments in the cerebral cortex nerve cells of senile and vitamin E deficient rats. *Acta Neuropath.* 9:7.

Nikaido, T.; Austin, J.; Rinehart, R.; Trueb, L.; Hutchison, J.; Stukenbrok, H.; and Miles, B. 1971. Studies in ageing of the brain. I. Isolation and preliminary characterization of Alzheimer plaques and cores. *Arch. Neurol.* 25:198.

Norton, W.T.; Poduslo, S.E.; and Suzuki, K. 1967. Rat brain myelin: Compositional changes during development. Abstract, Int. Soc. Neurochem., Strasbourg, p. 161.

Norton, W.T., and Poduslo, S.E. 1970. Neuronal soma and whole neuroglia of rat brain: A new isolation technique. *Science* 167:1144.

Oeriu, S. 1964. Proteins in development and senescence. In *Advances in Gerontological Research.* B.L. Strehler (ed.). New York: Academic Press, vol. 1, p. 23.

Ordy, J.M.; Samorajski, T.; Zeman, W.; and Curtis, H.J. 1967. Interaction effects of environmental stress and deuteron irradiation of the brain on mortality and longevity of C57BL/10 mice. *Proc. Soc. Exp. Biol. Med.* 126:184.

Ordy, J.M.; Samorajski, T.; Hershberger, T.J.; and Curtis, H.J. 1971. Life-shortening by deuteron irradiation of the brain in C57BL/10 female mice. *J. Geront.* 26:194.

Palade, G.E. 1955. Studies on the endoplasmic reticulum. II. Dispositions in cells *in situ. J. Biophys. Biochem. Cytol.* 1:567.

Palay, S.L., and Palade, G.E. 1955. The fine structure of neurons. *J. Biophys. Biochem. Cytol.* 1:69.

Pallis, C.A.; Duckett, S.; and Pearse, A.G.E. 1967. Diffuse lipofuscinosis of the central nervous system. *Neurology* 17:381.

Price, G.B.; Modak, S.P.; and Makinodan, T. 1971. Age-associated changes in the DNA of mouse tissue. *Science* 171:917.

Raine, C.S.; Poduslo, S.E.; and Norton, W.T. 1971. The ultrastructure of purified preparations of neurons and glial cells. *Brain Res.* 27:11.

Reichel, W. and Garcia-Bunuel, R. 1970. Pathologic findings in progeria: Myocardial fibrosis and lipofuscin pigment. *Amer. J. Clin. Path.* 53:243.

Retzlaff, E., and Fontaine, J. 1965. Functional and structural changes in motor neurons with age. In *Behavior, Aging, and the Nervous System.* A.T. Welford and J.E. Birren (eds.). Springfield, Ill.: Charles C Thomas, p. 340.

Ring, G.C.; Bosch, M.; and Lo, C.S. 1970. Effects of exercise on growth, resting metabolism and body composition of Fischer rats. *Proc. Soc. Exp. Biol. Med.* 133:1162.

Rouser, G., and Yamamoto, A. 1969. Lipids. In *Handbook of Neurochemistry.* A. Lajtha (ed.). New York: Plenum Press, vol. 1, p. 121.

Samorajski, T., and Friede, R.L. 1968. A quantitative electron microscopic study of myelination in the pyramidal tract of rat. *J. Comp. Neurol.* 134:323.

Samorajski, T.; Ordy, J.M.; and Rady Reimer, P. 1968. Lipofuscin pigment accumulation in the nervous system of aging mice. *Anat. Rec.* 160:555.

Samorajski, T.; Ordy, J.M.; Zeman, W.; and Curtis, H.J. 1970. Brain irradiation and aging. *Interdiscipl. Topics Gerontol.* 7:72.

Samorajski, T.; Friede, R.L.; and Ordy, J.M. 1971. Age differences in the ultrastructure of axons in the pyramidal tract of the mouse. *J. Geront.* 26:542.

Samorajski, T.; Rolsten, C.; and Ordy, J.M. 1971. Changes in behavior, brain, and neuroendocrine chemistry with age and stress in C57BL/10 male mice. *J. Geront.* 26:168.

Silberberg, M., and Silberberg, R. 1955. Diet and life span. *Physiol. Rev.* 35:347.

Smookler, H.H., and Buckley, J.P. 1969. Relationship between brain catecholamine synthesis, pituitary adrenal function and the production of hypertension during prolonged exposure to environmental stress. *Int. J. Neuropharmacol.* 8:33.

Strehler, B.L. 1960. Dynamic theories of aging. In *Aging. . . Some Social and Biological Aspects.* N.W. Shock (ed.). Washington, D.C.: American Association for Advancement of Science, p. 273.

Strehler, B.L. 1962. Aging of subcellular components. In *Time, Cells, and Aging.* B.L. Strehler (ed.) New York: Academic Press, p. 158.

Strehler, B.L., and Mildvan, A.S. 1962. Studies on the chemical properties of lipofuscin age pigment. In *Biological Aspects of Ageing.* N.W. Shock (ed.). New York: Columbia University Press, p. 174.

Strehler, B.L. 1966. Code degeneracy and the aging process: A molecular genetic theory of aging. In *Proceeding 7th International Congress of Gerontology.* Vienna: Viennese Medical Academy.

Sulkin, N.M., and Srivanij, P. 1960. The experimental production of senile pigments in the nerve cells of young rats. *J. Geront.* 15:2.

Sun, A., and Samorajski, T. 1970. Effects of ethanol on the activity of adenosine triphosphatase and acetylcholinesterase in synaptosomes isolated from guinea-pig brain. *J. Neurochem.* 17:1365.

Tauchi, H., and Sato, T. 1968. Age changes in size and number of mitochondria of human hepatic cells. *J. Geront.* 23:454.

Terry, R. 1963. The fine structure of neurofibrillary tangles in Alzheimer's disease. *J. Neurol. Exp. Neuropath.* 32:629.

Terry, R.; Gonatas, N.; and Weiss, M. 1964. Ultrastructural studies in Alzheimer's presenile dementia. *Amer. J. Path.* 44:269.

Tilney, R., and Rosett, J. 1931. The value of brain lipoids as an index of brain development. *Bull. Neurol. Inst.* (New York) 1:28.

Umaña, R., and Brekke, J.H. 1969. Changes in protease and ribonuclease activities in brain and liver during the life-span of the rat. *Growth* 33:157.

Várkonyi, T.; Domokos, H.; Maurer, M.; Zoltán, Ö.T.; Csillik, B.; and Földi, M. 1970. Die Wirkung von D,L-Kavain und Magnesium-Orotat auf die feinstrukturellen neuropathologischen Veränderungen der experimentellen lymphogenen Enzephalopathie. *Z. Geront.* 3:254.

Wisniewski, T.; Terry, R.; and Hirano, A. 1970. Neurofibrillary pathology. *J. Neuropath. Exp. Neurol.* 29:163.

Wulff, V.J.; Samis, H.V. Jr.; and Falzone, J.A. Jr. 1967. The metabolism of ribonucleic acid in young and old rodents. In *Advances in Gerontological Research*. B.L. Strehler (ed.). New York: Academic Press, vol. 2, p. 37.

Zeman, W., and Alpert, M. 1963. On the nature of the "stored" lipid substances in juvenile amaurotic idiocy. *Ann. Histochim.* 8:255.

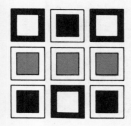

Neuropathology of Organic Brain Syndromes Associated with Aging

Nathan Malamud, M.D.

Laboratory of Neuropathology
Langley Porter Neuropsychiatric Institute
(California Department of Mental Hygiene)
and University of California
San Francisco, California

The organic brain syndrome is generally defined as a process of chronic progressive deterioration of cognitive, including memory, functions with secondary emotional, personality, and behavior disturbances. But while it has many different causes, its occurrence is most prevalent in association with the aging process.

Clinically, the diagnosis of senile or presenile dementia has been loosely applied to degenerative disorders that occur in advanced or middle age. Pathologically, they comprise distinct entities that are not to be confused even though at times they may coexist.

Table 1 lists the different types of pathology underlying the conditions under consideration, their incidence, range of age of onset, and sex distribution, as observed in a series of 1,225 autopsied cases.

Senile Brain Disease (SBD)

The pathology of SBD was first described in the latter part of the 19th and beginning of this century by a number of authors, notably Alzheimer, Perusini, and Simchowitz.

Grossly, the brain shows reduction in weight by approximately 5 to 17 percent, diffuse atrophy of the cerebral cortex, and compensatory dilatation of subarachnoid

NOTE: The opinions or conclusions stated in this paper are those of the author and are not to be construed as official or as necessarily reflecting the policy of the Department of Mental Hygiene.

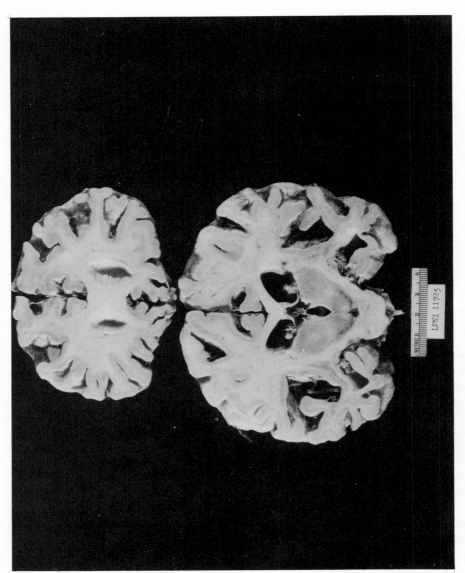

Figure 1. Coronal sections showing diffuse cerebral atrophy in a case of senile brain disease.

TABLE 1

Distribution of Types of Degenerative Disorders among 1,225 Cases

Type of Disorder	Age Range	No. of Cases	M/F Ratio
Senile brain disease	65 - 98	416 (34%)	3:2
Alzheimer's disease	40 - 64	103 (8.4%)	2:3
Pick's disease	35 - 72	35 (2.8%)	1:1
Creutzfeldt-Jakob's disease	43 - 86	32 (2.7%)	2:1
Arteriosclerotic brain disease	42 - 100	356 (29%)	2:1
Mixed senile-arteriosclerotic disease	62 - 94	283 (23%)	4:3

spaces and lateral ventricles (Figure 1). Microscopically, there is widespread decrease in cortical neurons with sclerosis and increased lipofuscin pigment in surviving nerve cells, accompanied by relatively mild astroglial response. The specific lesions on which the diagnosis rests are the presence of senile plaques, neurofibrillary tangles, and granulovacuolar changes. The plaques (Figure 2a) are spherical aggregates, from 5 to 150 μ in diameter, of either a filamentous to granular structure or with a dense central core that consists of a substance that is strongly argyrophilic, is variously positive for mucopolysaccharides and amyloid, and is birefringent with polarized light, associated with reaction by microglia and astroglia. Their most common location is in the cerebral cortex and hippocampal formation with much less tendency to occur in subcortical regions. The neurofibrillary tangles (Figure 2b) are characterized by proliferation of and conglutination of neurofibrils, resulting in bizarre shapes of neurons that are strongly argyrophilic, stain infrequently for amyloid, and show birefringence with polarized light. They likewise have a predilection for the hippocampal region and the cerebral cortex, especially the former. The granulovacuolar changes (Figure 2b) are intracytoplasmic argyrophilic granules surrounded by vacuoles that are virtually confined to the hippocampus. The interdependence of these three types of changes in SBD may be assumed from their constant association and staining reactions, although they differ in relative numbers and in regional predilection in different cases. It is, however, noteworthy that the neurofibrillary tangles and granulovacuolar changes may occur in the absence of senile plaques having been observed in a number of unrelated disorders such as in chronic encephalitis, in a unique degenerative disease occurring on the island of Guam, and occasionally in some other degenerative and metabolic diseases (Hirano and Zimmerman 1962). Specific vascular changes, other than coincidental arteriosclerosis, have been emphasized by some authors, such as capillary fibrosis (Gellerstedt 1933) and amyloid angiopathy (Scholz 1938).

The nature of the specific lesions in SBD has been much debated in the literature. The positive staining for amyloid has led Divry to look upon the condition as a primary amyloidosis (Divry 1952). In support of this view has been the demonstration by some

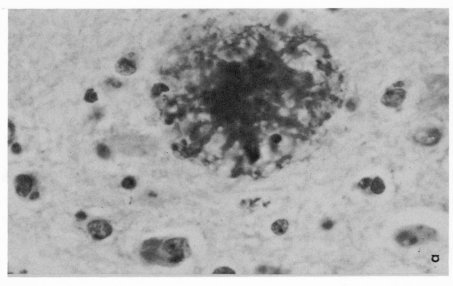

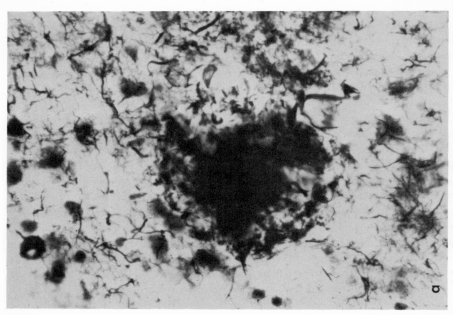

Figure 2. a, Senile plaque showing argyrophilic staining with Braunmühl's method, X 450 (left), and mucopolysaccharide content with periodic acid Schiff method, X 450 (right); (next page) b, neurofibrillary tangles (left) and granulovacuolar change (right) showing argyrophilia with Braunmühl's method, X 720.

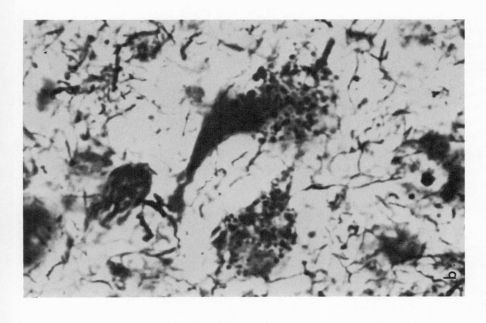

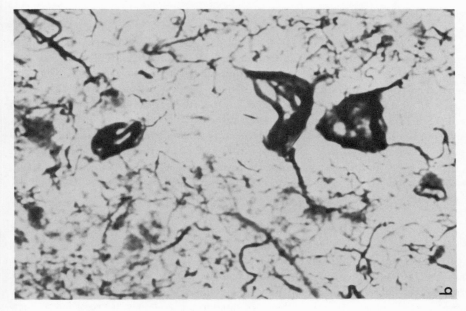

Figure 2b.

investigators (Vanderhorst, Stam, and Wigboldus 1960; Schwartz 1965) of similar amyloid deposits in various internal organs of senile patients. It is known, however, that the brain is an uncommon site for amyloid deposits in systemic amyloidosis. Even when this does occur, the deposit has a different distribution in the CNS, and only with rare exceptions does it take the form of senile plaques (Haberland 1964). Furthermore, the staining for amyloid has been inconstant as compared with the argyrophilia of the specific lesions. On the other hand, Braunmühl (1957) regarded the amyloid deposit in the brain as a secondary change, the primary condition, in his opinion, being a local condensation of the neuropil based on aging of colloids, a view that has been criticized recently by electron microscopists. At present electron microscopic and biochemical investigations have considerably broadened our knowledge of the nature of the senile process, and these will be discussed by others in this volume.

The importance given to the above-mentioned specific lesions in SBD as a substrate for the clinical picture has also varied from some who see them as the *sine qua non* underlying the dementia, to others who regard them as merely an expression of senescence. It is possible that the significance of the loss of neurons has been underestimated in the absence of quantitative studies of neuron populations, whereas counts of senile plaques and neurofibrillary tangles lend themselves more readily to clinicopathologic correlation.

Alzheimer's Disease (AD)

First described by Alzheimer in 1907, the disease has been considered by him as a form of presenile dementia because of occurrence at an earlier period of life, ranging between 40 and 65, of a pathologic condition similar to senile dementia. The term "presenile" has been criticized because, on the one hand, occasional cases with a much earlier age of onset have been reported, and, on the other, because the boundaries with senile dementia seem arbitrary. It would seem, rather, that acceptance of one designation, say Alzheimer's disease, would be preferable to apply to any condition having an identical pathologic substrate, regardless of the age of onset. Any attempts at delineation of clinical differences at different ages do not seem to be sufficiently precise or fruitful. Thus the cases of AD listed in Table 1 were distinguished from those of SBD only by their age of onset.

Pathologically, the changes in the brain of AD differ on the average from cases of SBD only in their somewhat greater intensity. Exactly the same gross picture of diffuse atrophy (Figure 3a) and microscopic features (Figure 3b) of senile plaques, neurofibrillary tangles, and granulovacuolar changes have also been noted. Arteriosclerotic changes are rare in AD as might be expected at an earlier age. Focal atrophies have been reported but they are uncommon and may be regarded as local accentuations of the process. With respect to etiology, familial occurrence has been recorded on occasion in AD but any genetic factor does not seem to be of a Mendelian kind. Various precipitating factors, such as trauma and toxic or infectious systemic disorders, have been reported in isolated cases but their etiologic significance remains obscure.

   Considerable interest has been aroused in recent years with increasing reports of the occurrence of pathologic changes of AD in elderly patients with Down's syndrome (Jervis 1948; Jelgersma 1958; Malamud 1964; Solitaire and Lamarche 1966; Olson and Shaw 1969). Examination of the brains of young mongoloid patients usually discloses stigmata of arrested development but no signs of atrophy (Figure 4a), by contrast with the gross cerebral atrophy and microscopic changes of AD in elderly mongoloids (Figures 4b, c, and d). In Table 2 a survey of the incidence of such changes in a series of cases of Down's

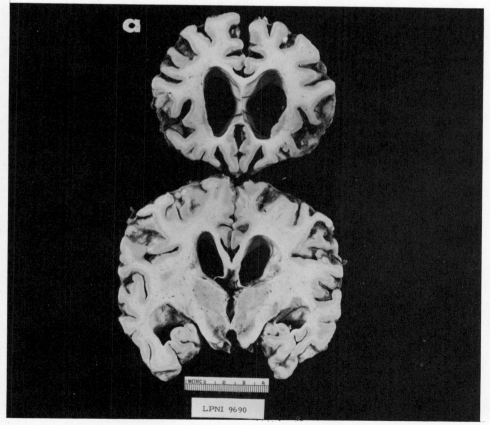

Figure 3. a, *Coronal sections illustrating diffuse cerebral atrophy in a case of Alzheimer's disease, showing in* (next page) b, *argyrophilic senile plaques and neurofibrillary tangles with Braunmühl's method. X 350.*

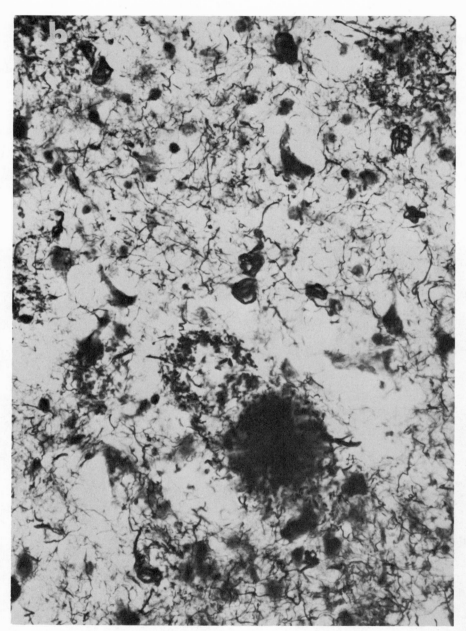

Figure 3b.

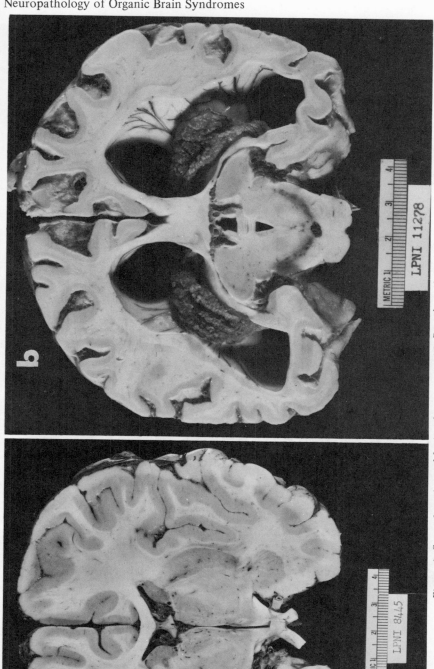

Figure 4. Coronal sections of brain of two cases with Down's syndrome as seen a, at a young age, showing nonspecific convolutional anomalies without signs of atrophy, and b, at middle age, demonstrating severe cortical atrophy, that in c and d (next pages) contains countless argyrophilic senile plaques and neurofibrillary tangles with Braunmühl's method. X 75 and 280.

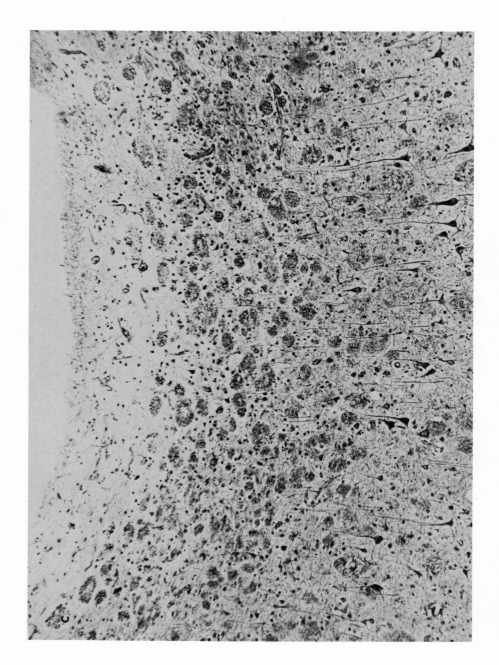

Figure 4c.

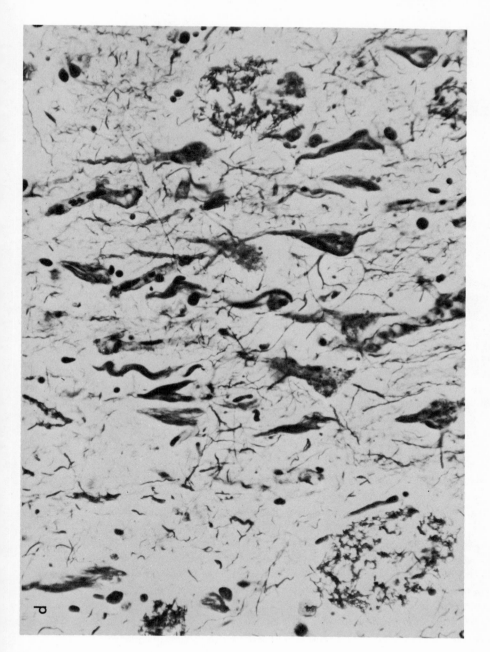

Figure 4d.

TABLE 2
Incidence of Alzheimer's Disease (AD) in 1,159 Cases of Mental Retardation (MR)

Type	Total No. Cases	Below Age 40	No. Cases with AD	Above Age 40	No. Cases with AD
MR with Down's syndrome	347	312	5 (1.6%)*	35	35 (100%)**
MR without Down's syndrome	813	588	0	225	31 (14%)***

  * Age range 20 to 38: all with mild changes of AD.
 ** Age range 42 to 69: 60% with severe, 40% with mild-moderate changes of AD.
*** Age range 54 to 86: all with mild changes of AD.

syndrome (DS) is compared with that in a miscellaneous group of mentally retardated cases without DS at approximately similar age periods. Of 347 cases with DS, 40 patients, ranging in age from 20 to 69 years at the time of death, showed pathologic changes typical of AD. They varied in intensity but in 60 percent they were unusually severe and comparable to the most advanced cases of AD. Furthermore, there were no patients with DS who lived past the age of 40 in whom such changes were not found. This was in marked contrast to their virtual absence in a series of 813 cases representing other forms of mental retardation, and even when found they were unusually mild, occurring only at very advanced age. The distribution of the AD changes in cases with DS, with respect to age and sex, is outlined in Table 3. It may be seen that, although only occasional and relatively mild changes were observed at ages below 40, in cases above age 40 there did not seem to be a linear distribution with advancing age since the changes were of almost equal intensity at all ages. As for the sex distribution, a ratio of 2 M : 3 F closely resembled that of the sex distribution of AD in the general population.

The clinical correlation of such brain pathology in patients with DS has not yet been adequately investigated. Only in isolated instances was there mention of mental deterioration or the development of seizures in adult mongoloids a few years prior to death. It is to be expected, of course, that the initially severe grade of mental retardation in DS is not conducive to adequate clinical evaluation. In a recent communication, Owens, Dawson, and Losin (1971) reported that clinical examination of 35 mongoloid subjects between the ages of 20 to 50 revealed no signs of gross dementia but subtle evidence of psychologic and neurologic deficit on comparison of the younger and older members of the group. Such studies, however, must be interpreted in the light of individual differences in the time of onset of AD.

The neuropathologic findings strongly suggest that the association of Down's syndrome and Alzheimer's disease is not fortuitous. As is well known, Down's syndrome is characterized by a variety of chromosomal abnormalities, such as trisomy 21, with or without mosaicism and dislocation. The relevance of these to the shorter life expectancy in the mongoloid has been discussed recently by Elam and Blumenthal (1970). The

TABLE 3
Age and Sex Distribution of Down's Syndrome with Alzheimer's Disease (AD)

Ages at Death	No. Cases	No. Cases with AD	Degrees of Changes	Ages at Death	Sex
First decade (birth - 10)	216	0	-	-	
Second decade (11 - 20)	49	1	1+	20	M1/F0
Third decade (21 - 30)	37	1	1+	21	M0/F1
Fourth decade (31 - 40)	10	3	3+	33, 37 and 38	M3/F0
Fifth decade (41 - 50)	15	15	4+ 2++ 9+++	(1 = 42; 3 = 43) (43, 49) (44 - 50)	M6/F9
Sixth decade (51 - 60)	15	15	4++ 11+++	(52, 53, 55, 56) (51 - 59)	M5/F10
Seventh decade (61 - 70)	5	5	1++ 4+++	(62) (61 - 69)	M1/F4
Total	347	40	9+ (22.5%) 7++ (17.5%) 24+++ (60%)	Range 20 - 69	M16 (40%) F24 (60%)

authors drew attention to the paradoxical association of various signs of delayed maturation and of premature aging in the mongoloid as, for example, in the late onset yet premature termination of maturation of bones, or in the late onset of menses but early development of the menopause, pointing to "a more rapid aging process in mongolism." It is likely that the same tendency is indicated in the initial signs of delayed brain development and the early occurrence of changes of Alzheimer's disease in Down's syndrome.

Elam and Blumenthal expressed the opinion that "longevity may be related to the ability of cells to maintain a stable chromosome state." In this respect, recent observations (Nielsen et al. 1968; Jarvik et al. 1971) seem to be relevant. These authors found a statistically significant increase of hypodiploid cells in female cases of senile dementia as compared with a control nondemented aged group. This suggested that the loss of chromosomes, due either to nondisjunction or chromosome lagging, was important in the etiology of senile dementia. Similar differences were, however, not observed in men. These findings are as yet based on small numbers of cases and their general import must await further confirmation.

Pick's Disease

It has been customary to include Pick's disease along with Alzheimer's disease as a form of "presenile dementia" on the assumption that it too represents premature aging. As a matter of fact, it was first described by Arnold Pick in 1892 as a form of senile dementia. It is a relatively rare disorder, occurring at about the same age range but not showing the female sex preponderance noted in Alzheimer's disease. Clinically, it is manifested by progressive dementia in which memory impairment is, however, not a feature, and by focal symptoms of aphasia, apraxia, and agnosia. Pathologically, Pick's disease is characterized grossly by sharply circumscribed areas of atrophy, involving bilaterally parts of frontal, temporal, and parietal lobes, singly or in combination (Figure 5a). The selection of areas of atrophy roughly corresponds to phylogenetically recently acquired cortical regions. Noteworthy is the virtual sparing of the hippocampal formation, to which the relative preservation of recent and retentive memory might be attributed as contrasted with impairment of this function in AD in which the hippocampus is consistently affected. Microscopically, neuronal loss is especially marked in supragranular cortical layers (Figure 5b) but the main difference from AD is the absence of senile plaques, neurofibrillary tangles, and granulovacuolar changes, and the presence of inflated neurons with or without intracytoplasmic argyrophilic inclusions (Figure 5c). Etiologically, evidence of a Mendelian dominant autosomal inheritance has been reported in a number of instances (Grünthal 1931; Sanders 1939; Malamud and Waggoner 1943; Sjögren 1952). But while the precise etiology remains obscure, the distinction from Alzheimer's disease is definite and the designation of "presenile" dementia to this condition is inappropriate.

Creutzfeldt-Jakob's Disease

This disorder has even less justification to be included with the "presenile" dementias, even though the age range is similar. First reported by Creutzfeldt in 1920 and more completely described by Jakob in 1921, it is a rare disorder. In fact, there has been some controversy with respect to its nosologic position (Nevin et al. 1960), yet it is increasingly becoming accepted as a clinicopathologic entity. The clinical course is generally rapid, varying from several months to a few years. It is characterized by progressive dementia associated with a great variety of motor and sensory disturbances involving pyramidal, extrapyramidal, cerebellar, lower motor neuron, and visual systems, in any combination. To this array of clinical manifestations correspond diffuse pathologic changes but with local predilection for either motor or sensory cortex, basal ganglia, cerebellum, cranial and/or spinal motor neurons. The gross changes in the brain are relatively inconspicuous, although in some instances there may be severe localized atrophy. The microscopic picture (Siedler and Malamud 1963) is dominated by a characteristic spongy type of degeneration, either laminar or diffuse, but without the specific lesions seen in the aforementioned conditions (Figure 6). Although the etiology remains unknown, recent attempts (Gajdusek and Gibbs 1969) to transmit the disease to chimpanzees has led the authors to speculate on a possible viral etiology. In any case, the

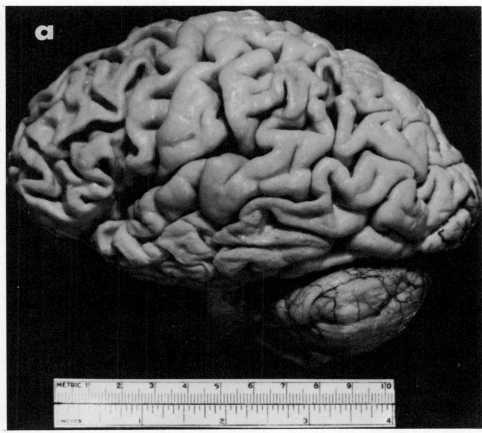

Figure 5. Lateral view in a case of Pick's disease, showing: a, circumscribed atrophy of parts of frontal, temporal and parietal lobes; (next pages) b, degeneration of supragranular layers of cortex, cresyl violet stain, X 140; and c, inflated neurons with cresyl violet stain, X 720 (top) and intracytoplasmic argyrophilic inclusions with Braunmühl's method, X 720 (bottom).

disorder has little in common with the presenile and senile dementias.

Hydrocephalic Dementia

Recent publications (Adams et al. 1965) have drawn attention to a syndrome characterized clinically by progressive dementia occurring in elderly individuals, associated with leg ataxia or spasticity, in which an occult or "low-pressure" hydrocephalus has been demonstrated by pneumoencephalography and in whom clinical recovery occurred following shunting procedures. The authors emphasized that the

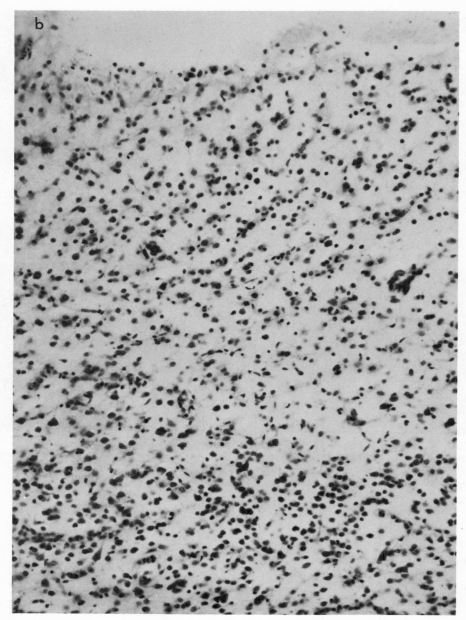

Figure 5b.

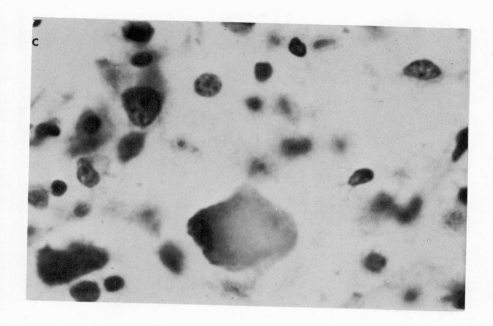

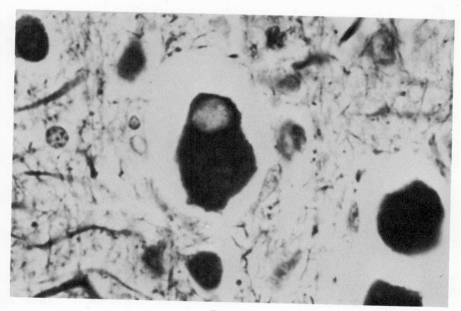

Figure 5c.

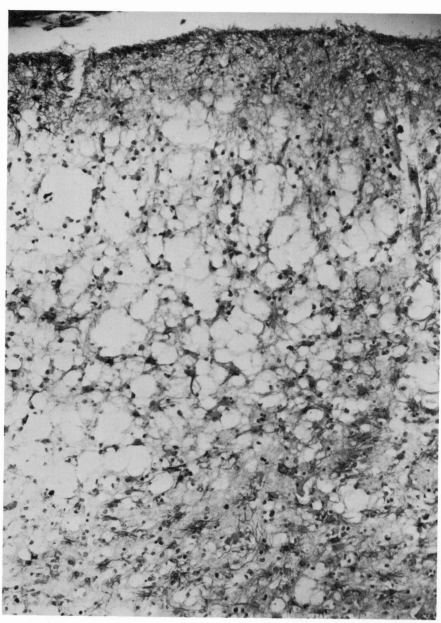

Figure 6. Case of Creutzfeldt-Jakob's disease, showing areas of spongy state and of astrogliosis in cerebral cortex with Holzer's glial method. X 120.

hydrocephalus was not related to brain atrophy, such as in the previously described conditions, but to obstruction in some part of the CSF circulation, although the exact site has not always been determined. But while it is well known that an arachnoiditis or stenosis of interventricular foramina, due to a variety of causes, can produce such a syndrome, nevertheless, the incidence of such a hopeful condition in the aging population is unfortunately low.

Arteriosclerotic Brain Disease (ASBD)

The role of vascular disease associated with cerebral and systemic arteriosclerosis, as a cause of dementia at advanced age, has long been recognized. It is believed, however, that its incidence has been overestimated, especially since a clinical differential diagnosis from other forms of chronic organic brain syndromes is often difficult. Fundamentally, the clinical features vary from the abrupt episodic occurrence in the form of strokes to more insidious and progressive expressions of derangement of cerebral circulation.

Since the pathologic findings were outlined in the beginning of the century (Alzheimer 1902) not much has been added. The vascular changes may be classified into (a) atherosclerosis of major and medium-sized vessels associated with infarcts in which there is complete tissue breakdown (Figures 7a and b), and (b) hyalinization of small blood vessels resulting in perivascular gliosis (Figure 7c) or other expressions of incomplete destruction. The great variety of lesions in size, age, and localization determines the clinical manifestations but it is not feasible to distinguish clearcut clinical forms.

Association of arteriosclerotic and senile brain disease is relatively common, sometimes one or the other predominating. From Table 1 it is apparent that pure cases of either SBD or ASBD are more common than their admixtures. It also seems obvious that the lack of interdependence of the two disease processes can be assumed in the face of exclusive occurrence of one or the other condition. The sex distribution bears out the general impression gained from the literature that ASBD is much more common in males than in females, although there is some male preponderance in all other categories at advanced age periods.

"Normal" Aging

For many years it had been accepted that senile and/or arteriosclerotic brain changes represent the substrate of the clinical picture of dementia. The validity of this concept has been questioned, however, since the demonstration by Gellerstedt in 1933 of the occurrence of similar brain changes in what he called "normal senile involution." Gellerstedt examined the brains of 50 patients, ranging in age from 65 to 97 years, who died in a general hospital from a variety of systemic diseases. All his cases were assumed to be mentally and neurologically normal although admittedly no detailed psychiatric examination had been performed. After excluding signs of vascular disease, he found in

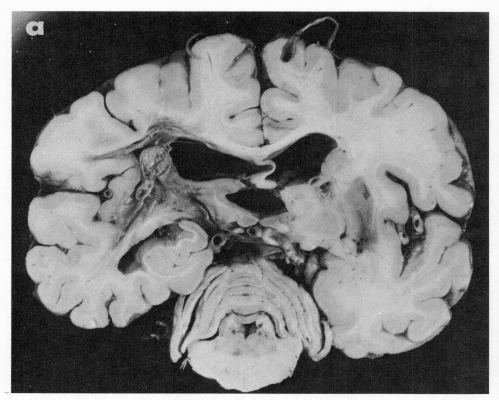

Figure 7. Case of cerebral atherosclerosis in a, coronal section showing severe atheromatous changes in major arteries associated with chronic infarcts and in (next pages) b, microscopic view of sclerotic blood vessels with adjacent cortical and subcortical old infarcts in a cystic stage: hematoxylin-van Gieson's method, X 5; c, case of arteriolar sclerosis of intracortical small blood vessels accompanied by focal perivascular gliosis: hematoxylin-eosin, X 100.

this group of "normals" all of the various gross and microscopic changes previously reported only in cases of senile dementia. Thus in 84 percent there were varying numbers of senile plaques in the cortex and in 82 percent neurofibrillary tangles that were, however, restricted to the hippocampal region. Gellerstedt concluded that the differences between "normal" and demented individuals were merely quantitative and that the senile plaques in particular were only manifestations of involution and not of disease.

Since then the clinical significance of the brain changes both in the causation of dementia and in relation to the aging process has been much discussed. Rothschild, in a

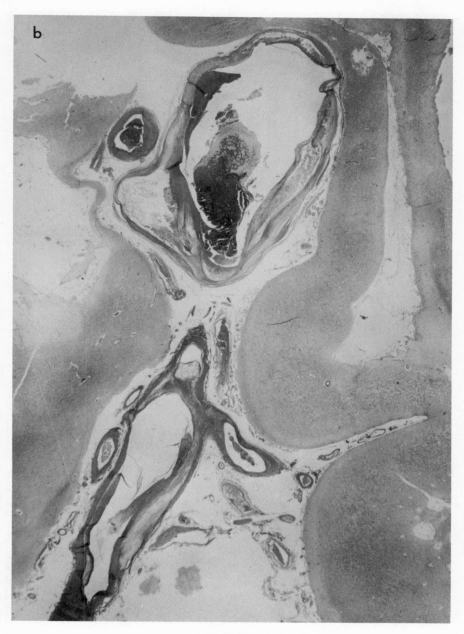

Figure 7b.

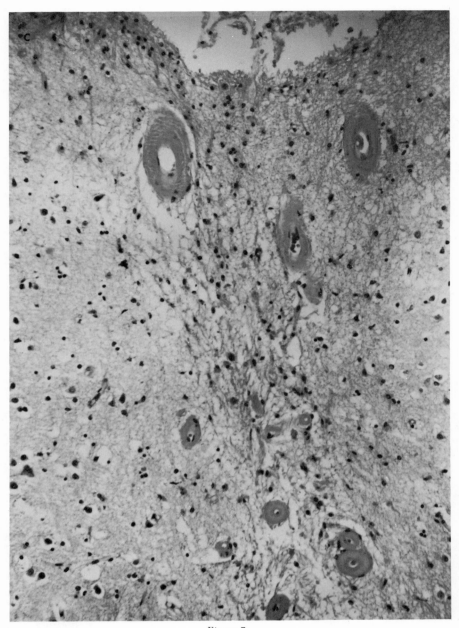

Figure 7c.

series of studies from 1937 to 1942 on small groups of either senile or arteriosclerotic psychosis, emphasized the lack of correlation between "extent of anatomic involvement and degree of intellectual deterioration," and stressed the greater importance of social and psychologic factors in the production of dementia. Corsellis (1960) took exception to such conclusions. He reported the findings in a series of 300 cases of elderly patients suffering from either an organic or functional disorder, and found in 75 percent of the organic group moderate to severe pathologic senile and/or arteriosclerotic brain changes, while in 75 percent of the functional group such brain changes were either absent or minimal. Simon and I (1965) reported similar pathologic differences between 220 cases of dementia, on the one hand, and 116 of functional disorders and 75 of "normal" individuals, on the other. We were especially impressed with the lack of or at most mild changes in the great majority of the "normals" by contrast with the experience of Gellerstedt.

It must be admitted that in all such studies precise clinical data were lacking in the groups of "normals" and functional disorders, and that the pathologic data were not based on exact quantitative estimates. More recent investigations have attempted to deal with some of these criticisms. Blessed, Tomlinson, and Roth (1968) compared the degree of intellectual deterioration as measured by a dementia score with mean senile plaque counts, extent of distribution of neurofibrillary tangles, and size of vascular lesions in a group of 50 demented, and in 28 control cases, aged 56 to 92 years. They found only quantitative differences between the two groups, so that in 70 percent of the demented cases the pathologic changes were much more severe than in any control case. Yet they admitted that further clinical investigations, especially more comprehensive psychologic studies, would be required to test the nondemented group with the more limited pathology. In a similar study, Dayan (1970) selected his "normal" control group among individuals who had no known history of prior illness and who died suddenly either as a result of trauma or unexpected ischemic heart attacks. In 47 such "normals" he found fewer than 40 percent who had senile plaques, neurofibrillary tangles, and granulovacuolar changes by contrast with a group of 40 cases of senile dementia, all of whom showed such lesions.

It would thus appear that while quantitative and not qualitative differences are thought to distinguish the demented from the normal population, the assumption that these changes represent mere variations in the physiologic aging process, which is only intensified in the dementias, is not yet substantiated. It is likely that the relatively mild changes in some of the nondemented individuals are clinically expressed in more subtle psychologic impairment that hitherto had not been precisely tested.

References

Adams, R.D.; Fischer, C.M.; Hakim, S.; Ojemann, R.G.; and Sweet, W.H. 1965. Symptomatic occult hydrocephalus with normal cerebrospinal fluid pressure. *New Eng. J. Med.* 273:117.

Alzheimer, A. (a) 1902. Die Seelenstörungen auf arteriosclerotischer Grundlage. *Allg. Ztschr. Psychiat.* 59:695. (b) 1907. Ueber eine eigenartige Erkrankung der Hirnrinde. *Allg. Ztschr. Psychiat.* 64:146.

Blessed, G.; Tomlinson, B.E.; and Roth, M. 1968. The association between quantitative measures of dementia and of senile changes in the cerebral gray matter of elderly subjects. *Brit. J. Psychiat.* 114:797.

Braunmühl, A. von 1957. Alterskrankungen des Zentralnervensystems. In *Handbuch der speziellen pathologischen Anatomie und Histologie.* O. Lubarsch, F. Henke, and R. Rössle (eds.). Berlin: Springer Verlag, vol. 13, p. 337.

Corsellis, J.A.N. 1962. *Mental Illness and the Aging Brain.* London: Oxford University Press.

Creutzfeldt, H.G. 1920. Ueber eine eigenartige herdförmige Erkrankung des Zentralnervensystems. *Ztschr. Neurol. Psychiat.* 56:1.

Dayan, A.D. 1970. Quantitative histological studies on the aged human brain. *Acta Neuropath.* 16:85.

Divry, P. 1952. La pathochimie générale et cellulaire des processus seniles et préseniles. In *Proceedings International Congress of Neuropathology, Rome.* Turin: Rosenberg and Sellier, vol. 2, p. 313.

Elam, L.H., and Blumenthal, H.T. 1970. Aging in the mentally retarded. In *Interdisciplinary Topics in Gerontology.* New York: S. Karger, vol. 7, p. 87.

Gajdusek, D.C., and Gibbs, C.J. 1969. Transmission of subacute viral encephalitides of man and animals. *Neurology* 19:291.

Gellerstedt, N. 1933. *Zur Kenntnis der Hirnveränderungen bei der Normalen Altersinvolution.* Uppsala: Almquist and Wiksells Boktryckeri-A-B.

Grünthal, E. 1931. Klinisch-genealogischer Nachweis von Erblichkeit bei Pickscher Krankheit. *Ztschr. Neurol. Psychiat.* 136:464.

Haberland, C. 1964. Primary systemic amyloidosis. *J. Neuropath. Exp. Neurol.* 23:135.

Hirano, A., and Zimmerman, H.M. 1962. Alzheimer's neurofibrillary changes. *Arch. Neurol.* 7:227.

Jakob, A. 1921. Über eigenartige Erkrankungen des Zentralnervensystems mit bemerkenswertem anatomischen Befunde. *Ztschr. Neurol. Psychiat.* 64:147.

Jarvik, L.F.; Altshuler, K.Z.; Kato, T.; and Blummer, B. 1971. Organic brain syndrome and chromosome loss in aged twins. *Dis. Nerv. Syst.* 32:159.

Jelgersma, H.C. 1958. Die frühzeitige Dementia senilis bei Mongoloiden. *Folia Psychiat. Neurol. Neurochir. Neerlandia* 61:367.

Jervis, G.A. 1948. Early senile dementia in mongoloid idiocy. *Amer. J. Psychiat.* 105:102.

Malamud, N. 1964. Neuropathology. In *Mental Retardation.* H.A. Stevens and R. Heber (eds.). Chicago: University of Chicago Press, p. 429.

Malamud, N., and Waggoner, R.W. 1943. Genealogic and clinicopathologic study of Pick's disease. *Arch. Neurol. Psychiat.* 50:288.

Nevin, S.; McMenemey, W.H.; Behrman, S.; and Jones, D.P. 1960. Subacute spongiform encephalopathy. *Brain* 83:519.

Nielsen, J.; Jensen, L.; Lindhardt, H.; Stottrup, L.; and Sondergaard, A. 1968. Chromosomes in senile dementia. *Brit. J. Psychiat.* 114:303.

Olson, M.I., and Shaw, C. 1969. Presenile dementia and Alzheimer's disease in mongolism. *Brain* 92:147.

Owens, D.; Dawson, J.C.; and Losin, S. 1971. Alzheimer's disease in Down's syndrome. *Amer. J. Ment. Def.* 75:606.

Pick, A. 1892. Ueber die Beziehungen der senilen Hirnatrophie zur Aphasie. *Prag. Med. Wochschr.* 17:165.

Rothschild, D. (a) 1937. Pathologic changes in senile psychoses and their psychobiologic significance. *Amer. J. Psychiat.* 93:757. (b) 1942. Neuropathologic changes in arteriosclerotic psychoses and their psychiatric significance. *Arch. Neurol. Psychiat.* 48:417.

Sanders, J.; Schenk, V.W.D.; and van Veen, P. 1939. *A Family with Pick's Disease.* Amsterdam: N.V. Noord-Hollandsche Vitgevers.

Scholz, W. 1938. Studien zur Pathologie der Hirngefässe. *Ztschr. Neurol. Psychiat.* 162:694.

Schwartz, P. 1965. Senile cerebral, pancreatic-insular and cardiac amyloidosis. *Trans. N. Y. Acad. Sci.* 27:393.

Siedler, H., and Malamud, N. 1963. Creutzfeldt-Jakob's disease. *J. Neuropath. Exp. Neurol.* 22:381.

Simon, A., and Malamud, N. 1965. Comparison of clinical and neuropathological findings in geriatric mental illness. In *Psychiatric Disorders in the Aged*. Manchester: Geigy (U.K.) Ltd., p. 322.

Sjögren, T. 1952. A genetic study of Morbus Alzheimer and Morbus Pick. In *Acta Psychiat. Neurol. Scandinav. Suppl. 82*. Copenhagen: Ejnar Munksgaard, p. 10.

Solitaire, G.B., and Lamarche, J.B. 1966. Alzheimer's disease and senile dementia as seen in mongoloids. *Amer. J. Ment. Def.* 70:840.

Vanderhorst, L.; Stam, F.C.; and Wigboldus, J.M. 1960. Amyloidosis in senile and pre-senile involutional processes of the central nervous system. *J. Nerv. Ment. Dis.* 130:578.

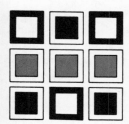

Ultrastructure of Senile Dementia and of Experimental Analogs

Robert D. Terry, M.D., and
Henryk M. Wiśniewski, M.D., Ph.D.

Department of Pathology (Neuropathology)
Albert Einstein College of Medicine
The Bronx, New York

The morphologic changes of age which concern the neuropathologist must be not only those he can correlate with clinical signs and symptoms, but also those he can relate to fundamental biology. It is the purpose of this paper to provide as much of this structural correlation as is currently possible in regard to Alzheimer's disease.

In our own experience, as well as that of most workers in the field, there are no significant differences between the most common form of senile dementia and the presenile type called Alzheimer's disease; throughout the rest of this chapter the terms will, therefore, be used synonymously. Adams and Sidman (1968) have stated that 80 to 90 percent of the patients institutionalized with organic dementia are probably afflicted with this form of disease. Considering that fact, as well as the great but uncountable number of those more or less disabled who are cared for at home, one can well recognize the enormous sociologic importance of this disease and its biologic background.

Its major macroscopic changes are cerebral atrophy, especially in the frontal region, and dilatation of the lateral ventricles. Since the turn of the century, two particular microscopic abnormalities, and several lesser ones, have been associated with Alzheimer's disease. These prime lesions are the neurofibrillary tangle of Alzheimer and the senile plaque. The other histologic findings include neuronal loss, lipofuscin accumulation, amyloid angiopathy, granulovacuolar degeneration and, most recently discovered, Hirano bodies.

Both the neurofibrillary tangle and the senile plaque are often seen in normal elderly patients. Matsuyama, Namiki, and Watanabe (1966) found the former in 81 percent of people autopsied in their seventh decade, and in 99 percent of those over 70 years old! The same authors noted senile plaques in 23 percent of those in the seventh

89

decade, and 68 percent of those in the ninth. The frequency of these lesions in the population as a whole, however, is not as pragmatically significant as to symptoms as is their concentration in any given case. In the normal aged population, therefore, there is a discrepancy between the morphological findings and the mental preservation for which there would seem to be three explanations which probably operate together. First, the brain is usually thought to be structurally redundant, with a considerable amount of spare circuitry, especially in some cortical areas. Second, there are many silent areas of the cerebrum in which quite large lesions can be placed without their being accompanied by overt symptoms. And third, our ability to test for subtle brain alterations is still quite crude. Roth, Tomlinson, and Blessed (1966), in a prospective study of the aged, found a high degree of positive correlation between the frequency of plaques and psychometric deficiency as measured by a battery of tests. Therefore, these lesions, although present in the normal elderly, cannot be regarded as merely incidental as to mental disease of this type.

At the Einstein College of Medicine, beginning in 1962 in collaboration with the late Dr. Saul R. Korey, we have had the opportunity to study 18 brain biopsies of histologically verified Alzheimer's disease or senile dementia of this type (Terry, Gonatas, and Weiss 1964; Terry and Wiśniewski 1970; Terry 1971). We have also examined a series of very aged dogs (Wiśniewski et al. 1970), and a single rhesus monkey (Wiśniewski and Terry 1972) which was about 24 years old and showed signs of advanced aged. There were striking similarities among these specimens and significant species differences that bear intensive questioning. All tissue was studied light microscopically by means of the usual aniline dyes and Bodian preparations. Furthermore, tissue fixed with glutaraldehyde and subsequent osmic acid was embedded in plastic and sectioned at a thickness of one micron, stained with toluidine blue, and examined with the light microscope. This stain technique was found to be extraordinarily revealing and permitted ready correlation between light and electron microscopy. The dogs and the monkey were perfused *in vivo* through the heart with paraformaldehyde, followed by glutaraldehyde. After dissection of the brain, selected portions were fixed with osmic acid, dehydrated in ethanol, and embedded according to the usual techniques in epoxy resin.

Spontaneous Lesions

The neurofibrillary tangle (Figure 1) was found (Kidd 1963; Terry 1963) ultrastructurally to be composed of bundles of extraordinary fibrillar elements present, to date, only in human material. These abnormal structures measure about 220 Å at their widest, and are constricted at about 800 Å intervals to a width of about 100 Å (Figure 2). A clear space is readily seen between the walls in the wider regions. Cross sections have two distinct appearances, the interpretations of which are not yet clear. With about equal frequency are seen, on the one hand, crescentic forms sometimes with a granule in the concavity, and on the other hand are circular forms whose wall is granular and about 50 Å in thickness (Figure 3). According to the latter cross sections, these elements making up the neurofibrillary tangle have been interpreted as constricted or twisted

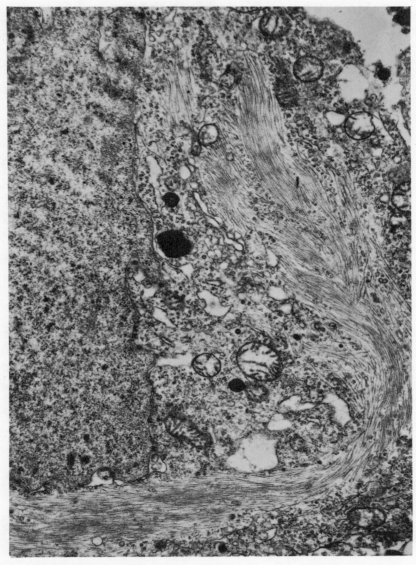

Figure 1. An electron micrograph of a human cortical neuron with a neurofibrillary tangle coursing through the cytoplasm. The tangle is made up principally of numerous abnormal twisted elements. The nucleus is present at the left. Cytoplasmic elements are essentially normal. X 12,000.

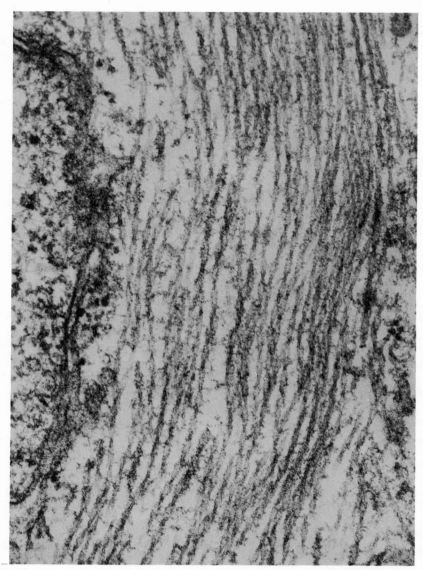

Figure 2. Higher magnification of the "twisted tubules" comprising a neurofibrillary tangle in another neuron. The twist occurs every 800 Å, the maximum width is about 200 Å, and the minimum width about 100 Å. Some delicate side branches are evident. X 75,000.

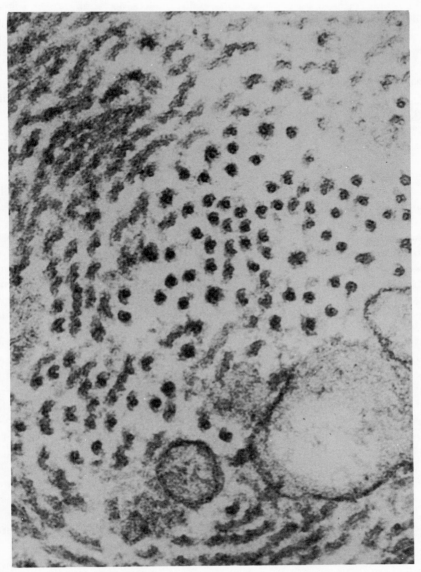

Figure 3. Cross sections of the elements of a neurofibrillary tangle reveal both crescentic and circular configurations. Some of the latter are seen to contain a fine central core. X 165,000.

tubules (Terry 1963; Hirano et al. 1968), but following the lead of the crescentic cross sections, Kidd (1963) described them as bifilar helices. Isolation studies (Shelanski, Liwnicz, and Slusarek 1971) by techniques of differential centrifugation have not yet clarified this problem. Bundles of these "twisted tubules" course through the cytoplasm of the affected neuronal soma, displacing and replacing the organelles normally found in this location. Mixed with the twisted tubules are recently found, smooth-walled tubules. Normal, smooth microtubules whose outer diameter is 240 Å are quite rare in these cells. Lipofuscin of the usual compound appearance is often, but by no means invariably, found in the neurons with neurofibrillary tangles. The other organelles in the perikaryon appear to be quite unremarkable.

One would very much like to know whether the protein that composes these twisted tubules is a new one, or a modified normal protein. In the latter case, we would think that normal microtubule protein has possibly been oxidized, perhaps by a failure of the antioxidation system. If, for example, sulfhydril or methionine groups were oxidized to disulfides periodically along the microtubule, its configuration could change to this regularly twisted shape. It is known (Hallgren and Sourander 1960), incidentally, that the affected brains have abnormally high concentrations of iron, which could act as the oxidizing agent. But should these abnormal tubules be found to be made up of an entirely new protein, one would have to consider a slow virus or a previously repressed gene now acting on the cell's protein-synthesizing apparatus. In regard to the latter suggestion, it should be noted that familial cases of Alzheimer's disease are quite common (Feldman et al. 1963). As to slow viruses, it is to be pointed out that neurofibrillary tangles of this configuration are found in the pigmented neurons of the brain stem in cases of postencephalitic Parkinsonism which follow Von Economo's lethargic encephalomyelitis (Wiśniewski, Terry, and Hirano 1970). Although the Guam-Parkinsonism-Dementia complex has not yet been proved to be viral in nature, this etiology, coinciding probably with a genetically controlled susceptibility, is a strong possibility. In that bizarre condition, found only among the Chamorro Indians native to the Mariana Islands, great numbers of cerebral neurons contain neurofibrillary tangles, again composed of these twisted tubules (Hirano 1970). The neurofibrillary degeneration described in conjunction with subacute sclerosing panencephalitis (Krücke 1961) has not yet been studied electron microscopically. Neither have those apparently similar lesions found in the cerebrum of patients with Down's syndrome (Olson and Shaw 1969), which are often associated with a visible chromosomal abnormality indicating obvious genetic disturbance. It is clear, then, that studies to determine the nature of the twisted tubule are of prime importance. Some such studies are under way in our laboratory.

While the spontaneous neurofibrillary tangle made up of abnormal fibrillar material has, to date, been found only in human beings, the senile plaque, which would seem to be better called the neuritic plaque, can be studied in dogs and monkeys as well (Wiśniewski and Terry 1972). As seen in the electron microscope, the plaque has a complex structure with three major components—abnormal neurites, amyloid, and glial cells (microglia, macrophages, and astrocytes). The prominence of each of these elements determines the light microscopic appearance of the plaque, and variations have given rise to three major classes of plaque—primitive, classical, and burned out or compact (Figures 4, 5, and 6).

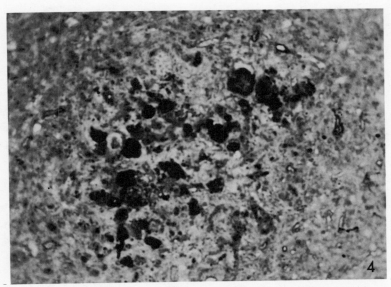

Figure 4. A one-micron thick, plastic-embedded section stained with toluidine blue reveals a primitive senile plaque made up of strongly and weakly stained neurites, and without an amyloid core. Reproduced with permission from the Ciba Foundation Symposium on Alzheimer's Disease and Related Conditions, *page 148. X 560.*

The smallest lesion in the neuropil that we have found with the electron microscope, and the one we therefore believe to be the earliest precursor, is an abnormal neurite, invisible to the light microscopist by itself or even in a small group. It is larger than normal and packed with mitochondria which are minimally shrunken and distinctly granular and dense, relative to the normal (Figure 7). Their cristae are slightly swollen. Laminated dense bodies are also present in these abnormal neurites. In the presence of one, two, or three of these neurites in a particular area, amyloid is usually absent. However, when there are larger clusters of such neurites, then, ultrastructurally, amyloid is almost invariably present in the form of intercellular wisps of typical amyloid fibrils. This small cluster, made up primarily of degenerating neurites with a few wisps of amyloid and perhaps a microglial cell, is recognizable with the light microscope as a primitive plaque, as named by von Braunmühl (1957) (Figure 8).

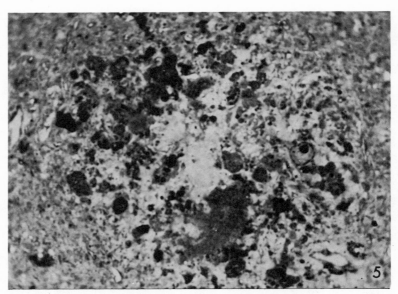

Figure 5. *A classical or typical plaque, with central core of amyloid surrounded by corona of deeply colored neurites, stained with the same methods. Reproduced with permission from the* Ciba Foundation Symposium on Alzheimer's Disease and Related Conditions, *page 148. X 560.*

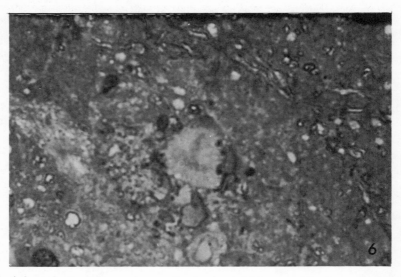

Figure 6. *A burned-out plaque made up of a large amyloid core, without surrounding neurites. Reproduced with permission from the* Ciba Foundation Symposium on Alzheimer's Disease and Related Conditions, *page 148. X 560.*

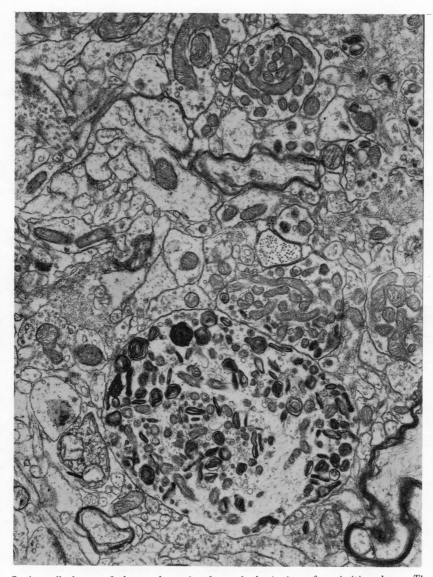

Figure 7. A small cluster of abnormal neurites forms the beginning of a primitive plaque. They are crowded with abnormally dense mitochondria, and, in the case of the larger one below, also contain dense bodies. A little extracellular amyloid is present in this early lesion. X 15,000.

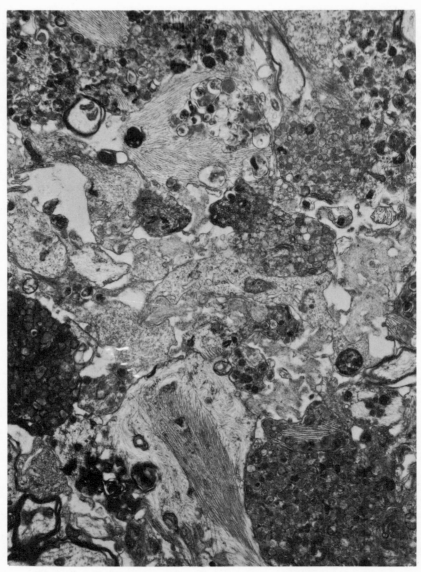

Figure 8. Another primitive plaque, somewhat further along in development, is made up of many enlarged neurites packed with dense bodies and bundles of twisted tubules. Small wisps of amyloid are present in the extracellular space. X 4,500.

If one can be permitted to draw sequential inferences from this large series of photomicrographs, the next stage reveals a compact central core of amyloid, sometimes with star-shaped radiations, surrounded by a zone of neurites containing degenerating mitochondria, dense bodies, and abnormal fibrillar material. This complex is the classical plaque (Figure 9). The dense bodies in the neurites are often laminated, with a periodicity of 40 to 45 Å, and have been shown to contain acid phosphatase (Suzuki and Terry 1967). They therefore are in the lysosome series of cytoplasmic organelles. Transitional forms between mitochondria and the dense bodies are commonly noted, and this probably occurs by means of a process of autophagy. Macrophages are frequently involved in these plaques. They contain chiefly complex lipid forms resembling lipofuscin and lesser amounts of cellular debris. Not infrequently these macrophages also contain within their cytoplasm amyloid fibrils, probably in the process of being extruded into the extracellular space to form the core. The abnormal fibrillar material in the neurites is identical to that present in the neuronal perikaryon where it makes up the neurofibrillary tangle. It is wholly absent from the otherwise identical plaques of the dogs and the monkey.

Glenner and his colleagues (1971) have recently noted that amyloid is made up of a polymer of light chains of immunoglobulin. He has proposed that, following some antigenic stimuli, there is an excess of light chains, which enter the lysosomes, become partially degraded, and are then polymerized usually in the extracellular space in the form of amyloid. Intracellular amyloid is thought to form when there is a great excess of substrate (Zucker-Franklin and Franklin 1970). However, the reason for the amyloid being present in Alzheimer's disease is by no means clear. Elderly patients, whether they have Alzheimer's disease or not, almost invariably have some degree of vascular amyloidosis. It seems quite possible that in the presence of this systemic amyloidosis, the microglia, as members of the reticuloendothelial system, are also "tuned up" for amyloid synthesis. When they are attracted to the plaque by the degenerating neurites, they are switched on to local amyloid production as well as to phagocytosis, since the synthetic apparatus is already available. In this context the amyloid component of the plaque might be considered as simply coincidental. It is more difficult to explain the presence of amyloid in the relatively youthful cases of Alzheimer's disease. Here one might postulate that whatever causes the neurites to degenerate also causes the reticuloendothelial system to produce amyloid.

The third type of plaque is compact, and may be considered as burned out, as it is composed primarily of a large mass of amyloid. There may be microglia, macrophages, or astrocytic processes around it, but degenerating neurites have by now disappeared (Figure 10).

The cause of the degeneration of the neurites is the critical problem at this time. It is possible that in Alzheimer's disease, where the neuronal soma is seriously affected by neurofibrillary tangles, diminished axoplasmic flow induces a dying-back phenomenon in the terminals of the axis cylinders. It is important to recall that one of the two major

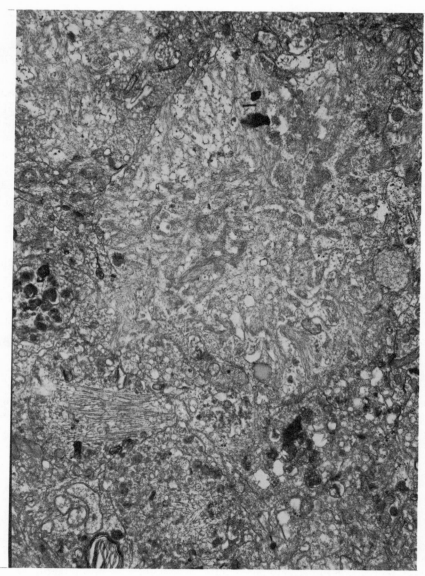

Figure 9. A mature typical plaque has a central core of amyloid surrounded by a corona of enlarged
neurites containing dense bodies, degenerating mitochondria, and abnormal microtubules. Microglia
are not visible at this level. X 4,000.

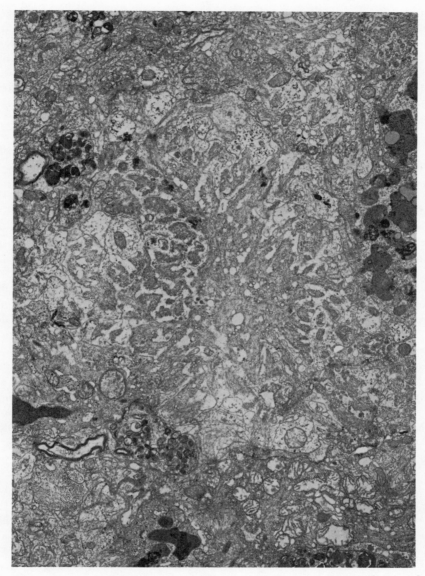

Figure 10. This is a small, burned-out or compact plaque, with a dense core of amyloid surrounded by macrophages containing lipid and astrocytic processes containing glycogen. Neurites have almost disappeared. X 4,000.

functions of microtubules (the other being the support of asymmetric structure) is to promote cytoplasmic flow, that is, axoplasmic flow as far as the nervous system is concerned (Porter 1966). This has been amply demonstrated by experiments in which tubules are dispersed by spindle inhibitors, and axoplasmic flow is halted (Karlsson, Hansson, and Sjöstrand 1971). It would seem that where normal microtubules are replaced by abnormal elements such as twisted tubules, the axoplasmic flow might similarly be abnormal and perhaps inadequate. It is conceivable that masses of lipofuscin within the perikaryonal cytoplasm might also be responsible for the degeneration of the terminals. Such lipofuscin accumulations are of course common in the elderly.

It should be noted, however, that abnormal tubules need not be related at all since, in the Guam-Parkinsonism-Dementia complex, there are many neurofibrillary tangles, and plaques are rare. The opposite side of the coin is represented by that type of case in which plaques are found and neurofibrillary tangles are absent. We have noted such plaques in a single biopsy of Pick's disease (Wiśniewski, Coblentz, and Terry 1971), and perhaps even more significant are the common plaques in the senile dogs and monkey in which neurofibrillary tangles in the neuronal soma and twisted tubules in the plaque are wholly absent.

Along with senile plaques and neurofibrillary tangles, we have found numerous secondary lesions which can readily be correlated with those long known to light microscopists. Myelin deterioration is noteworthy and undoubtedly accounts at least in part for the shrinkage of the centrum semiovale and the hydrocephalus ex vacuo. The alterations of the myelin sheath are of two types. We have seen examples of Wallerian degeneration in which the axis cylinders are broken up and granular, with subsequent degeneration of the surrounding myelin sheaths. We have also found examples of an unexpected type of primary demyelinization (Terry, Gonatas, and Weiss 1964) in which the axon is apparently intact, while the surrounding myelin is undergoing obvious degeneration (Figure 11). This is by no means specific to this disorder; we have also seen it in a few biopsies of Creutzfeldt-Jakob disease (Gonatas, Terry, and Weiss 1965) and various other cerebral biopsies.

While autopsy material is not usually satisfactory for electron microscopy, it is sometimes the only way in which one can get at certain structures like the human hippocampus which are inaccessible to the usual brain biopsy. Granulovacuolar change is found in the neurons of Ammon's horn, in this relatively poorly preserved material, to be a vacuole bounded by a unit membrane containing clear material and a core of finely granular, highly insoluble, dense matter (Figure 12). This corresponds to a typical autophagic body in which we would expect a small quantity of acid hydrolases.

The eosinophilic structure which is now known by his name was only recently discovered by Hirano and his colleagues (1968) in Guam-Parkinsonism-Dementia complex material. He soon thereafter found it to be present also in Alzheimer's disease, and this has been confirmed by many observers. The structure of the Hirano body has not yet

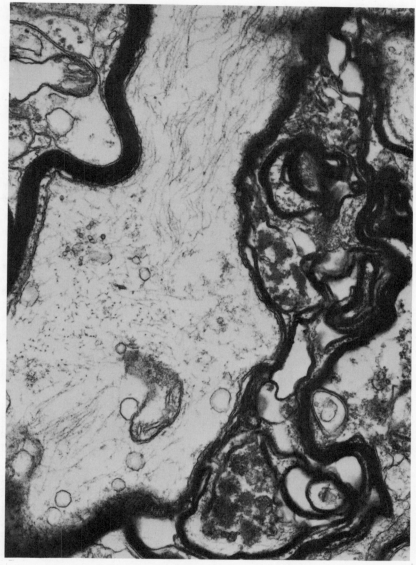

Figure 11. A normal axis cylinder, containing the usual complement of fibrillar material and mitochondria, is surrounded by degenerating myelin sheaths. Granular debris and myelin ovoids lie among the myelin lamellae. This must be defined as primary demyelinization. X 20,400.

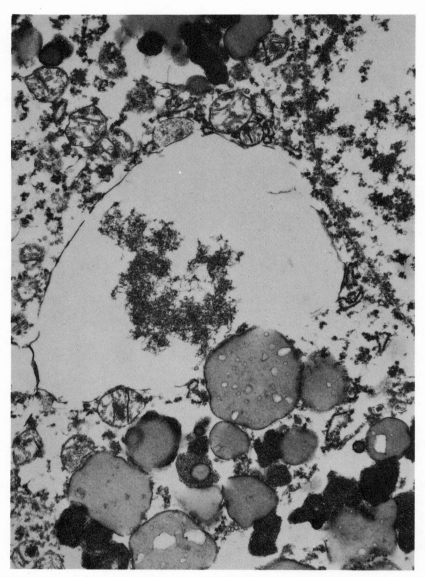

Figure 12. This is granulovacuolar degeneration of Simchowicz as seen by electron microscopy of an autopsied hippocampal neuron. The limiting membrane is artifactitiously disrupted. The adjacent cytoplasm is also poorly preserved, but lipofuscin is prominent. X 12,000.

been resolved in three dimensions, but it appears to be a paracrystalline material perhaps in the form of alternating sheets and rows of fibers (Figure 13). The significance of the structure is wholly unknown, but it is not impossible that it represents a crystallization of

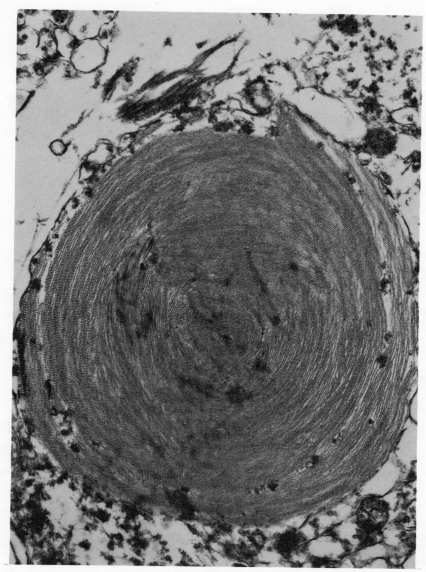

Figure 13. This is a cross section of a Hirano body from autopsy material. Where the crystal is cut perpendicular to its long axis, the membrane and filament structure can be distinguished. In the tangential regions it appears to have a herringbone or cross-hatched appearance. X 22,400.

the protein making up the twisted tubules.

Congophilic angiopathy is seen to involve primarily the perithelial cells and basement membrane. The latter structure is widened and replicated by the presence of masses of amyloid fibrils. These bundles not infrequently protrude into the adjacent parenchyma where they elicit no apparent reaction from the nearby neurites. Sometimes, however, there are paravascular plaques which abut on this vascular amyloid. This substance was relatively sparse in the plaques of the senile dog, but where the plaques were found in a paravascular location, the amyloid was indeed more prominent between the degenerating neurites.

We may summarize the preceding as follows: Human beings, dogs, and monkeys spontaneously develop senile neuritic plaques. Only the human being develops neurofibrillary tangles, and the human plaques differ from those of the other animals by the absence, in the latter, of the twisted tubules that characterize the perikaryonal tangles. The substructure of Alzheimer's disease may be delineated as follows:

Dementia: Neuronal and neuropil loss; tangles; synaptic changes.
Cortical atrophy: Neuronal and neuropil loss.
White matter atrophy: Wallerian and primary demyelinization.
Neurofibrillary tangles: Aggregated abnormal tubules.
Senile Plaques:
  Argentophilia: Complex lipid and lipofuscin; neurofibrillar aggregates in neurites.
  Congophilia: Amyloid extra- and intracellular.
  Excess hydrolytic and oxidative activity: Dense bodies and mitochondria in neurites.
Granulovacuolar degeneration: Autophagic bodies.
Hirano bodies: Fibrillar mat.
Congophilic angiopathy: Amyloid in basement membrane and adjacent parenchyma.

Experimentally Induced Lesions

In about 1954, Klatzo (personal communication, 1962) noted a curious vacuolar change in rabbit neurons when the animals were treated intrathecally or intracerebrally with small amounts of aluminum hydroxide or Holt's adjuvant. A few years later it was discovered by the current authors, at that time working separately, that these vacuoles were in actuality filled with neurofibrillar material (Klatzo, Wiśniewski, and Streicher 1965; Terry and Peña 1965). The affected neurons, which were present especially in the brain stem and spinal cord regardless of the site of injection, displayed changes similar to those of human neurofibrillary tangles when stained with the Bodian technique. Higher resolution electron microscopic analyses, however, demonstrated that the tangles were composed of filamentous elements rather than twisted tubules (Figures 14 and 15). These

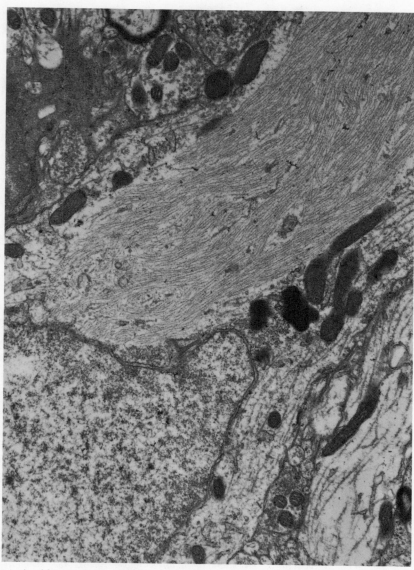

Figure 14. A rabbit anterior horn cell treated with aluminum salt. A filamentous neurofibrillary tangle occupies much of the cytoplasm, but normal microtubules are also present in the cytoplasm. X 12,000.

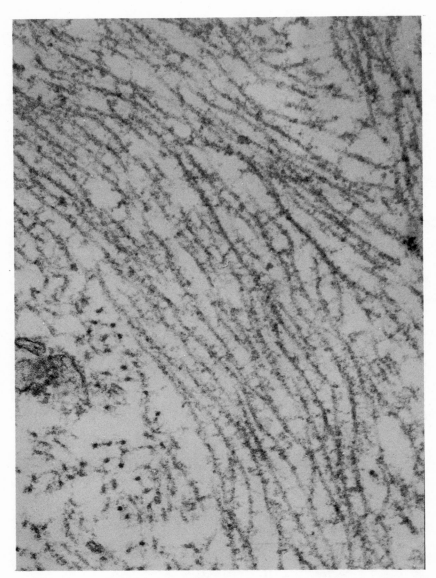

Figure 15. Higher magnification of an aluminum-induced tangle reveals the elements to be filamentous, measuring about 100 Å in width. There is an inconspicuous lumen in each filament, while short, delicate, perpendicular branches or cross bridges are quite obvious. Cross section of these filaments at the upper left confirms their circular configuration. X 100,000.

filaments were apparently identical to normal neurofilaments, being 100 Å in diameter and displaying short, thin, perpendicular side arms and poorly demarcated lumen (Wiśniewski and Terry 1970; Wiśniewski, Terry, and Hirano 1970). Theorizing that whatever the fine structure of the tangle, the essential functional abnormality was interference with axoplasmic flow, we hypothesized that a longer term experiment (the usual study was only two weeks) would reveal not only neurofibrillary tangles but also senile plaques in these rabbits, which were, incidentally, young adults. This proved to be the case, and a few plaques were indeed demonstrated in chronic animals (Figure 16A and B). These lesions were sparse and were incomplete relative to the human lesion in that they lacked the amyloid core as well as twisted tubules. They did, however, display typical degenerating neurites, filaments, and mitochondria (Figures 17 and 18). Rabbits and cats have been utilized so far in these experiments, and we have not yet been able to combine experimental amyloidosis with experimental plaques.

Some years ago Gonatas and Robbins (1964) recognized that treatment of the intermitotic HeLa cell with the spindle inhibitor colchicine caused an apparent increase in the cytoplasmic microfilaments. Peterson and Murray (1966) later noted a toxic effect in cultured neurons when they were similarly treated. Our own studies demonstrated that this drug induced proliferation of neurofibrils. These effects have been tested extensively in many laboratories both *in vivo* and *in vitro*, utilizing primarily colchicine, vincristine, and vinblastine (Wiśniewski, Shelanski, and Terry 1968). These compounds are known to cause the depolymerization of spindle tubules and their analogs; that is, microtubules in general and neurotubules in particular. Intrathecal treatment of rabbits with very low doses of either compound induces many neurofibrillary tangles and the disappearance of neurotubules in the neurons of the central nervous system. The filaments making up the tangle are morphologically (but possibly not chemically) identical to normal filaments, and the aggregates are quite similar to those found after treatment with aluminum salts. However, while in the latter case the other organelles of the neuron remain normal, this is not true following treatment with one of the spindle inhibitors. Here we find that the nuclear membrane has increased porosity, that mitochondria are clustered, that there is a decrease in the membranous component of the endoplasmic reticulum, and that autophagic bodies form within the cytoplasm seemingly from the rough endoplasmic reticulum (Figure 19). After treatment with vinblastine, large crystals made up of microtubule protein appear in the neuronal cytoplasm (Schochet, Lampert, and Earle 1968), and these as well as the tangles (Shelanski and Wiśniewski 1969) have also been found in human beings treated with vinblastine for lymphoma. The crystals have been duplicated *in vitro* by the addition of vinblastine to solutions of microtubule protein (Bensch et al. 1969). This system, as a matter of fact, is the basis for the quantitative precipitation of microtubule protein in an analytic technique recently described by Marantz, Ventilla, and Shelanski (1969). When the dose is small and the animals are carefully nursed, they often recover from their paresis within a few days, and microtubules reappear in great numbers within the cytoplasm. The nerve roots are of interest at this moment in the experiment because the fibers of the dorsal root are completely normal, since the dorsal root ganglion neurons are unaffected, while the axons

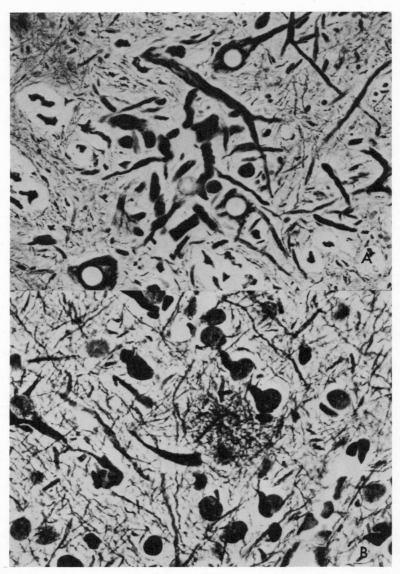

Figure 16 A and B. Senile plaques found in the rabbit long after treatment with aluminum, stained by the Bodian technique. Amyloid was not present. Reproduced with permission from the Ciba Foundation Symposium on Alzheimer's Disease and Related Conditions, *page 231. X 560.*

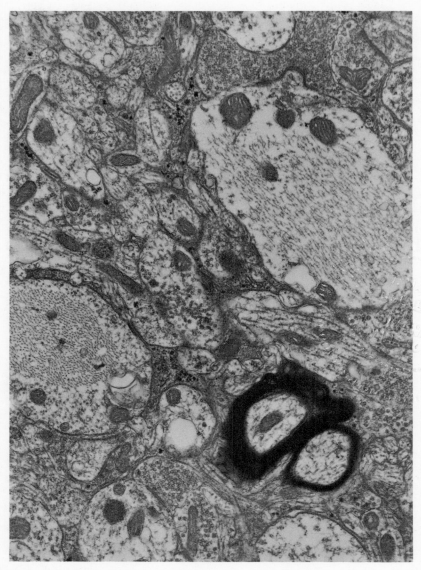

Figure 17. Electron micrograph of a rabbit plaque induced by aluminum shows several neurites filled with filamentous bundles. X 13,500.

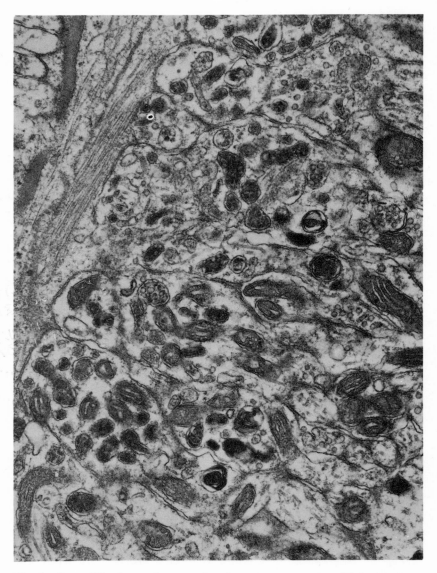

Figure 18. Another rabbit plaque demonstrating the numerous neurites filled with degenerating mitochondria and dense bodies. X 20,400.

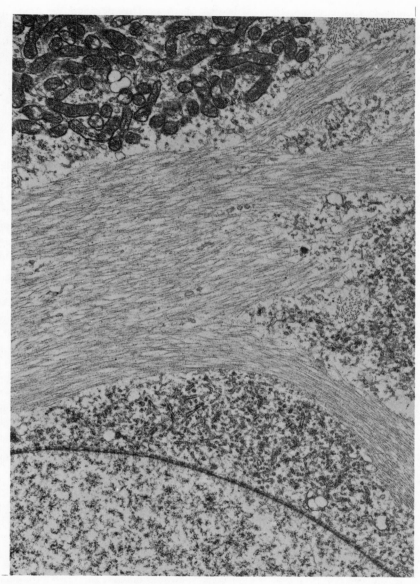

Figure 19. A rabbit neuron affected by treatment with colchicine. The nuclear membrane below demonstrates numerous pores; the mitochondria are clumped; the endoplasmic reticulum has lost much of its membranous component, and there is an obvious large tangle made up of filamentous elements. Reproduced with permission from Archives of Neurology *20:205, 1969. X 10,000.*

of the anterior root are undergoing obvious necrosis. This degeneration takes place despite the recovery of the spinal motor neurons from which the degenerating axons have come. This demonstrates that fatal changes in the axon can be associated with a transient loss of microtubular function within the neuronal soma. The mechanism for this degeneration is presumed to be interruption of axoplasmic flow, since it is known that the spindle inhibitors affect cytoplasmic movement as they depolymerize the microtubules (Karlsson, Hansson, and Sjöstrand 1971).

We can only speculate at this time about the relationship between these phenomena and those found in the aging human brain. It does, however, seem reasonable that diminished axoplasmic flow, for whatever reason, might well be responsible for at least some of the neuritic degeneration that is at the heart of senile plaque formation. Plaques and tangles occur independently in the human being, and the one appears routinely without the other in aged dogs and monkeys. Their pathogenesis must, therefore, be considered separately. Nevertheless, since the lesions are so often associated in the human being, and since a logical connection between the abnormal fibrillar material and diminished axoplasmic flow can be made so readily, inferences as to a causal relationship are tempting.

Two problem areas can clearly be delineated in this major disease. One has to do with neural fibrous protein as to the neurofibrillary tangle. The other is synaptic pathology in reference to senile plaques.

Acknowledgments

We are grateful to Ms. Loyda Menez, Lawrence Gonzales, and Sidney Gravney for their expert technical assistance. Ms. R.E. Butler's editorial assistance is much appreciated.

This work was supported in part by grants NS 02255 and NS 03356 from the National Institutes of Health.

Dr. Wiśniewski is a Career Scientist of the Health Research Council of the City of New York, Grant No. I-679.

References

Adams, R.D., and Sidman, R.L. 1968. *Introduction to Neuropathology.* New York: The Blakiston Division, McGraw-Hill Book Company, p. 511.
Bensch, K.G.; Marantz, R.; Wiśniewski, H.; and Shelanski, M. 1969. Induction in vitro of microtubular crystals by vinca alkaloids. *Science* 165:495.
Braunmühl, A.v. 1957. Alterserkrankungen des Zentralnervensystems. Senile Involution. Senile Demenz. Alzheimersche Krankheit. In *Handbuch der Speziellen Pathologischen Anatomie und Histologie*, XIII. Part 1. A. Erkrankungen des zentralen Nervensystems 1:337. O. Lubarsch, F. Henke, and R. Rössle (eds.). Berlin: Springer Verlag.

Feldman, R.G.; Chandler, K.A.; Levy, L.L.; and Glaser, G.H. 1963. Familial Alzheimer's disease. *Neurology* 13:811.

Glenner, G.G.; Terry, W.; Harada, M.; Isersky, C.; and Page, D. 1971. Amyloid fibril proteins: Proof of homology with immunoglobulin light chains by sequence analyses. *Science* 172:1150.

Gonatas, N.K., and Robbins, E. 1964. The homology of spindle tubules and neuro-tubules in the chick embryo retina. *Protoplasma* 59:25.

Gonatas, N.K.; Terry, R.D.; and Weiss, M. 1965. Electron microscopic study in two cases of Jakob-Creutzfeldt disease. *J. Neuropath. Exp. Neurol.* 24:575.

Hallgren, B., and Sourander, P. 1960. The non-haemin iron in the cerebral cortex in Alzheimer's disease. *J. Neurochem.* 5:307.

Hirano, A. 1970. Neurofibrillary changes in conditions related to Alzheimer's disease. In *Ciba Foundation Symposium on Alzheimer's Disease and Related Conditions.* G.E.W. Wolstenholme and M. O'Connor (eds.). London: J. & A. Churchill, p. 185.

Hirano, A.; Dembitzer, H.M.; Kurland, L.T.; and Zimmerman, H.M. 1968. The fine structure of some intraganglionic alterations. Neurofibrillary tangles, granulovacuolar bodies and "rod-like" structures as seen in Guam amyotrophic lateral sclerosis and Parkinsonism-Dementia complex. *J. Neuropath. Exp. Neurol.* 27:167.

Karlsson, J.-O.; Hansson, H.-A.; and Sjöstrand, J. 1971. Effect of colchicine on axonal transport and morphology of retinal ganglion cells. *Z. Zellforsch.* 115:265.

Kidd, M. 1963. Paired helical filaments in electron microscopy of Alzheimer's disease. *Nature* 197:192.

Klatzo, I.; Wiśniewski, H.; and Streicher, E. 1965. Experimental production of neurofibrillary degeneration. I. Light microscopic observations. *J. Neuropath. Exp. Neurol.* 24:187.

Krücke, W. 1961. Chronic sclerosing "leucoencephalitis and polyneuritis with intranuclear inclusion bodies." In *Encephalitides. Proceedings of a Symposium on the Neuropathology, Electroencephalography and Biochemistry of Encephalitides,* Antwerp 1959. L. Van Bogaert, J. Radermecker, H. Hozay, and A. Lowenthal (eds.). Amsterdam: Elsevier Publishing Company, p. 560.

Marantz, R.; Ventilla, M.; and Shelanski, M. 1969. Vinblastine-induced precipitation of microtubule protein. *Science* 165:498.

Matsuyama, H.; Namiki, H.; and Watanabe, I. 1966. Senile changes in the brain in the Japanese. Incidence of Alzheimer's neurofibrillary change and senile plaques. In *Proceedings of the 5th International Congress of Neuropathology.* F. Luthy and A. Bischoff (eds.). *Excerpta Medica* Series No. 100, p. 979.

Olson, M.I., and Shaw, C.-M. 1969. Presenile dementia and Alzheimer's disease in mongolism. *Brain* 92:147.

Peterson, E., and Murray, M. 1966. Serial observations in tissue cultures on neurotoxic effects of colchicine. *Anat. Rec.* 154:401 (abstr.).

Porter, K.R. 1966. Cytoplasmic microtubules and their functions. In *Ciba Foundation Symposium on Principles of Biomolecular Organization.* G.E.W. Wolstenholme and M. O'Connor (eds.). Boston: Little, Brown, p. 308.

Roth, M.; Tomlinson, B.E.; and Blessed, G. 1966. Correlation between scores for dementia and counts of "senile plaques" in cerebral grey matter of elderly subjects. *Nature* 209:109.

Schochet, S.S., Jr.; Lampert, P.W.; and Earle, K.M. 1968. Neuronal changes induced by intrathecal vincristine sulfate. *J. Neuropath. Exp. Neurol.* 27:645.

Shelanski, M.L.; Liwnicz, B.H.; and Slusarek, W. 1971. Biochemical studies on Guam Parkinsonism Dementia. *Trans. Amer. Assoc. Neuropath.* San Juan, P.R., June 1971. P. 36.

Shelanski, M.L., and Wiśniewski, H. 1969. Neurofibrillary degeneration induced by vincristine therapy. *Arch. Neurol.* 20:199.

Suzuki, K., and Terry, R.D. 1967. Fine structural localization of acid phosphatase in senile plaques in Alzheimer's presenile dementia. *Acta Neuropath.* 8:276.

Terry, R.D. 1963. The fine structure of neurofibrillary tangles in Alzheimer's disease. *J. Neuropath. Exp. Neurol.* 22:629.

Terry, R.D. 1971. Presidential address. Neuronal fibrous protein in human pathology. *J. Neuropath. Exp. Neurol.* 30:8.

Terry, R.D., Gonatas, N.K.; and Weiss, M. 1964. Ultrastructural studies in Alzheimer's presenile dementia. *Amer. J. Path.* 44:269.

Terry, R.D., and Peña, C. 1965. Experimental production of neurofibrillary degeneration. 2. Electron microscopy, phosphatase histochemistry and electron probe analysis. *J. Neuropath. Exp. Neurol.* 24:200.

Terry, R.D., and Wiśniewski, H.M. 1970. The ultrastructure of the neurofibrillary tangle and the senile plaque. In *Ciba Foundation Symposium on Alzheimer's Disease and Related Conditions.* G.E.W. Wolstenholme and M. O'Connor (eds.). London: J. & A. Churchill, p. 145.

Wiśniewski, H.M.; Coblentz, J.M.; and Terry, R.D. 1971. Pick's disease. A clinical and ultrastructural study. *Arch Neurol.* (in press).

Wiśniewski, H.; Johnson, A.B.; Raine, C.S.; Kay, W.J.; and Terry, R.D. 1970. Senile plaques and cerebral amyloidosis in aged dogs. A histochemical and ultrastructural study. *Lab. Invest.* 23:287.

Wiśniewski, H.; Shelanski, M.L.; and Terry, R.D. 1968. Effects of mitotic spindle inhibitors on neurotubules and neurofilaments in anterior horn cells. *J. Cell Biol.* 38:224.

Wiśniewski, H.; and Terry, R.D. 1970. An experimental approach to the morphogenesis of neurofibrillary degeneration and the argyrophilic plaque. In *Ciba Foundation Symposium on Alzheimer's Disease and Related Conditions.* G.E.W. Wolstenholme and M.O'Connor (eds.). London: J. & A. Churchill, p. 223.

Wiśniewski, H.M.; and Terry, R.D. 1972. Reexamination of the pathogenesis of the senile plaque. In *Progress in Neuropathology.* vol. 2. H.M. Zimmerman (ed.). New York: Grune & Stratton (in press).

Wiśniewski, H.; Terry. R.D.; and Hirano, A. 1970. Neurofibrillary pathology. *J. Neuropath. Exp. Neurol.* 29:163.

Zucker-Franklin, D., and Franklin, E.C. 1970. Intracellular localization of human amyloid by fluorescence and electron microscopy. *Amer. J. Path.* 59:23.

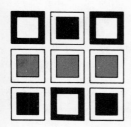

Cerebral Physiology of the Aged: Influence of Circulatory Disorders

Walter D. Obrist, Ph.D.

Duke University Medical Center
Durham, North Carolina

The Concept of Cerebrovascular Insufficiency

The purpose of this paper is to examine the concept of vascular insufficiency as it relates to cerebral physiologic alterations in old age and to associated states of intellectual deterioration. Vascular insufficiency has been defined as an inadequate blood supply relative to the metabolic needs of the tissue (Sokoloff 1961). It may be present continuously or occur intermittently whenever blood flow falls below normal levels, or it may become manifest only under conditions of increased metabolic demand.

Hemodynamically, vascular insufficiency develops when tissue perfusion pressure drops in relation to vascular resistance. The resulting decrease in blood flow may then give rise to ischemic hypoxia. Cerebrovascular insufficiency, which is analogous to coronary insufficiency, has been produced experimentally in animals by reductions in blood pressure following arterial ligation (Corday, Rothenberg, and Putnam 1953; Denny-Brown and Meyer 1957). The severity of the resulting EEG, neurological, and pathological changes depends on the magnitude of the blood pressure decline, the degree of vessel stenosis, and the adequacy of collateral circulation. Clinically, it has been suggested that cerebrovascular insufficiency may account for episodic focal neurological signs in cases with no demonstrable vascular occlusion (Denny-Brown 1960; Zülch 1969). Both apoplectic and transient ischemic attacks have been attributed to acute drops in blood pressure. Recent evidence, however, suggests that fluctuations in blood pressure only occasionally precipitate such episodes (Kendell and Marshall 1963; Fazekas and Alman 1964; Millikan 1965; Drake and Drake 1968), which are now believed to be primarily of thromboembolic origin (Paulson 1971).

Although cerebrovascular insufficiency may contribute little to episodic

117

neurological disturbances, a question arises concerning the extent to which it can account for age-related changes in mental function. It is conceivable that subacute, prolonged, or intermittent ischemia (with resulting hypoxia) may produce diffuse degenerative changes in the brain which lead to behavioral and intellectual impairment. Acute hemostasis and tissue infarction need not be the only consequence of cerebrovascular insufficiency; in fact, such dramatic events might be exceptions that occur only when a hemodynamic crisis reaches catastrophic proportions. Rather, it seems likely that the usual effects of ischemic hypoxia are more subtle, involving histologic, ultrastructural, and cytochemical changes (Schadé and McMenemey 1963). Impairment of higher integrative functions would depend on the widespread cerebral distribution of such effects and their accumulation over time. The concomitant occurrence of anemia or pulmonary insufficiency, both prevalent in old age, could easily exacerbate the underlying hypoxia.

A major difficulty with the concept of cerebrovascular insufficiency is that the phenomenon is not amenable to direct observation. The neurologist has been understandably reluctant to infer insufficiency states in the absence of objective neurological or radiological evidence. Such a cautious approach, however, has had the consequence of restricting the concept of cerebrovascular insufficiency to conditions manifested by focal neurological signs. The psychiatrist, on the other hand, has been more prone to infer vascular insufficiency on the basis of mental changes, even though he lacks adequate criteria for making such a judgment.

Psychological studies of stroke have emphasized the relationship between discrete cognitive deficits and localized encephalopathy (Meier 1970). There is some evidence, however, that circulatory disorders other than cerebrovascular accidents can affect mental function in senescence. Significant correlations have been reported between intellectual impairment, which is usually generalized, and clinical evidence of various diseases involving the cardiovascular system (Obrist et al. 1962; Birren et al. 1963; Szafran 1963; Spieth 1964; Jalavisto 1964/65; Kezdi et al. 1965; Eisdorfer 1967; Reitan 1970; Wilkie and Eisdorfer 1971; Busse and Wang 1972). Thus, middle-aged and elderly subjects with heart disease, hypertension, reduced pulmonary function, peripheral arteriosclerosis, and transient cerebrovascular symptoms showed greater intellectual decline than those with minimal or no evidence of such disorders. Unfortunately, the precise nature of the pathophysiology in these cases was not determined. These findings nevertheless point to the possible role of cerebrovascular insufficiency in the development of intellectual deterioration in old age and emphasize the need for evaluating the status of the cerebral circulation.

The present paper will attempt to review those aspects of cerebral physiology that have relevance to senescent mental function. Before describing some of the physiological findings, the question might be asked whether there is any morphological basis for assuming that cerebrovascular disease is related to senile intellectual changes.

Vascular Disease and the Dementias of Old Age

In a recent paper on dementia in cerebrovascular disease, Fisher (1968) described several conditions in which intellectual deficit accompanies specific vascular pathology, including strokes, bilateral stenosis of the carotid arteries, and multiple lacunar infarcts. He argued that "cerebrovascular dementia is a matter of strokes large and small," and that such disorders should be distinguished from Alzheimer's disease, in which senile plaques and neurofibrillary changes predominate. Unfortunately, the neurological and psychiatric examinations are not always capable of making such an easy differentiation, especially in patients in whom the two types of pathology coexist. Several extensive morphological investigations that shed some light on this problem are now available on aged mental hospital patients.

Malamud (1965) and Simon and Malamud (1965) found that 68 percent of 220 patients with organic brain syndrome had multiple areas of cerebral softening which the authors attributed to arteriosclerosis. Of these, more than one third had little or no evidence of senile brain disease (i.e., plaques and neurofibrillary tangles), while the remainder showed such changes to a variable degree. Comparable cerebral softenings were found in only 20 percent of elderly control subjects. Similar findings have been obtained by Tomlinson, Blessed, and Roth (1970), who observed a quantitative relationship between the amount of cerebral softening and the severity of intellectual deficit. Fifty cubic centimeters or more of necrotic tissue were found in 32 percent of patients with organic brain syndrome, an amount encountered in only 7 percent of an elderly control group. A significant number of senile plaques was observed in about half of the demented patients, but when plaques and softening occurred together, it was the latter that accounted for most of the variance in intellectual function (Roth 1971).

The lower than expected incidence of significant cerebral softening lead Tomlinson and coworkers (1970) to conclude that "arteriosclerotic dementia is almost certainly overdiagnosed clinically." Although probably correct, this argument assumes that infarct necrosis is the only manifestation of ischemic hypoxia. Microscopic lesions consisting of widespread acellular areas and extensive gliosis commonly result from cerebral ischemia (Bailey 1963), and they may occur independently of gross tissue softening in patients with cerebrovascular disease (Rothschild 1942). Similar microscopic changes in the absence of gross focal destruction have been observed in the brains of patients with cardiac insufficiency (Riggs and Wahal 1962). Unlike senile plaques, such lesions are difficult to identify and quantify but nevertheless need to be considered in assessing the effects of cerebral ischemia.

Observations on vessel pathology are equally difficult to quantify. Using a four-point scale, Corsellis (1962) rated the severity of both macroscopic and microscopic vascular changes in the brains of 300 elderly mental hospital patients and correlated them with parenchymal lesions. Moderate-to-severe large vessel atherosclerosis and small vessel degeneration were observed in approximately 50 percent of patients with organic brain syndrome, in whom they were twice as prevalent as in patients with functional psychosis. Some overlap between vascular changes and senile plaques was noted, the latter occurring in about one third of the demented patients. An interesting finding in the Corsellis study was the high incidence of death due to heart disease in the demented group, an observation also made by Rothschild (1942). This suggested to both authors the possibility that systemic circulatory disturbances may contribute to pathological changes in the brain.

From the few morphological studies available, it may be concluded that cerebrovascular disease is an important factor in the etiology of certain types of dementia. The question is not whether vascular disease is capable of producing dementia, which seems well established, but rather to what extent it can account for the prevalence of this disorder in old age. A similar question might be raised about the milder intellectual changes occurring in normal senescence, where considerable neuronal depopulation has been found (Brody 1955 and 1970). Because postmortem observations are limited to the end-point of a disease process, they contribute little to an understanding of its evolution during life. The physiological investigations described below are aimed at a better understanding of intellectual deterioration as it develops in the elderly person.

The EEG and Circulatory Disorders in Senescence

Electroencephalographic findings in old age and their relationship to physical and mental status are the subject of a recent comprehensive review (Obrist 1972) and will only be summarized here. The major age-related EEG change in senescence is a slowing down of the dominant alpha rhythm from a mean frequency of approximately 10 cps (cycles per second) to 8 or 9 cps. The magnitude of this slowing has been found to be significantly related to health status, longevity, and intellectual function. Thus, aged individuals who remain healthy and active show only minor EEG deviations from young-adult norms, while those with various chronic illnesses, particularly circulatory disorders, undergo decreases in alpha frequency. As in the case of young adults, EEG findings bear little or no relationship to intelligence test performance in healthy old subjects in whom both alpha frequency and cognitive function are well-preserved. Significant correlations between EEG and mental function are obtained, however, in subjects with clinically evident diseases of the cardiovascular system, where alpha frequency and intelligence test performance undergo parallel declines (Obrist et al. 1962).

Figure 1 illustrates two types of EEGs commonly found in elderly community volunteers. The upper tracing shows a 10-cps alpha rhythm in a normal subject who continues in good health at the present time, eleven years later. The lower tracing reveals a diffusely slow alpha rhythm of 8 cps mixed with occasional 6- to 7-cps theta waves. This subject, who suffered from severe heart disease, but was compensated at the time of recording, died 18 months following his EEG. A postmortem examination revealed advanced coronary sclerosis and arteriolonephrosclerosis; gross cerebral findings were unremarkable.

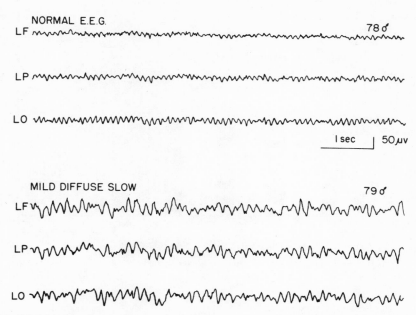

Figure 1. EEG recordings from two elderly community volunteers. Upper tracing: A 10-cps alpha rhythm in a healthy 78-year-old man. Lower tracing: Mixed alpha and theta activity in a 79-year-old man with severe heart disease. LF, LP, LO = left frontal, parietal, and occipital areas, respectively. All leads are referred to the homolateral ear.

Nonfocal alpha slowing occurs in patients with circulatory disorders regardless of whether the disease is manifest in the heart, periphery, or brain. Figure 2 compares the alpha frequency of 46 residents of an old age home who had normal and abnormal electrocardiograms (Obrist and Bissell 1955). Alpha frequency was significantly slower in the subjects with electrocardiographic abnormalities. All of the subjects with abnormal EKGs had a clinical history of heart disease with impaired functional capacity, but only two showed signs of congestive heart failure at the time of EEG recording. Eight of the subjects with abnormal EKGs had, in addition, focal neurological signs suggestive of cerebrovascular disease. Alpha slowing in these cases was also nonfocal, and no greater than in those with cardiac symptoms only.

The above findings can be interpreted in a number of ways. There is evidence that cerebral blood flow is reduced in heart failure (Scheinberg 1950b; Eisenberg, Madison, and Sensenbach 1960) and that it is quantitatively related to cardiac output (Shapiro and Chawla 1969). Abnormally slow EEGs have also been observed in heart failure (Ewalt and Ruskin 1944), where the degree of slowing is correlated with cerebral blood flow (Sulg et al. 1969). Since a slow alpha rhythm was found in cardiac patients who were compensated, it seems unlikely that acute heart failure with associated reductions in cerebral blood flow can account for more than a few of the observed EEG changes.

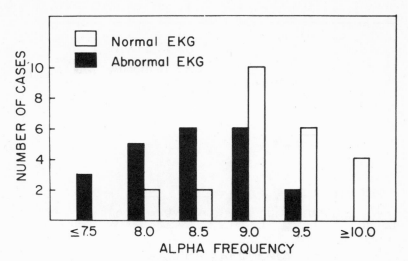

Figure 2. Alpha frequency in 46 age-matched residents of a retirement home who had normal and abnormal electrocardiograms (EKG). Mean age = 77 years. The groups differ significantly in alpha frequency at the .01 level.

It is quite possible, of course, that no direct causal relationship exists between heart disease and EEG. The apparent correlation may simply reflect a high concordance between coronary and cerebrovascular disease (Young et al. 1956; Kannel 1971), the latter being the critical variable. A more plausible explanation, however, is that repeated episodes of reduced cardiac output, either alone or in combination with cerebrovascular disease, result in transient states of cerebral ischemia which have cumulative and irreversible effects on the EEG. This hypothesis, although a reasonable one, requires confirmation.

The EEG shows more pronounced alterations in aged patients with organic brain syndrome (Obrist 1972). Slow waves in the theta (4 to 7 cps) and delta (1 to 3 cps) bands usually predominate, appearing bilaterally and diffusely over the head. Both the degree of diffuse slowing and the extent of its spatial distribution are related to the severity of intellectual deterioration. This is in sharp contrast to the focal slow activity commonly found over the temporal area in normal elderly subjects, which bears little or no relationship to mental status, including learning and memory function. Because diffuse slow activity is correlated with mental deterioration, its absence or presence has permitted a rough differentiation between functional and organic psychoses in old age.

.Some years ago, the author and coworkers observed a relationship between blood pressure and the incidence of diffuse slow activity in a heterogeneous group of aged psychiatric patients (Obrist, Busse, and Henry 1961). The upper graph in Figure 3 illustrates this finding, which was based on 233 hospitalized patients and 261 elderly community controls. Whereas few of the control subjects had diffusely slow EEGs,

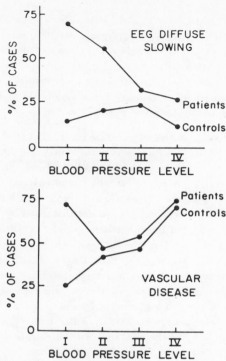

Figure 3. Upper graph: *Incidence of diffuse EEG slow activity (less than 7 cps) at four blood pressure levels in two groups of elderly subjects — 233 hospitalized psychiatric patients and 261 community controls. Lower graph: Incidence of clinically detectable vascular disease plotted against blood pressure level in the same subjects. Blood pressure subgroups were formed by dividing the respective samples into four equal parts, based on mean arterial pressure. Subjects with malignant hypertension were excluded.*

almost half of the psychiatric patients revealed this type of tracing, the highest incidence occurring at the lower blood pressure levels. Patients with elevated pressures, on the other hand, showed less diffuse slowing, a finding consistent with the observations of Harvald (1958) and Turton (1958). Tranquilizer intake in a few of the subjects could not explain the results.

The observed relationship between EEG and blood pressure in aged psychiatric patients suggested the occurrence of cerebrovascular insufficiency, that is, low blood pressure in the presence of increased vascular resistance leading to a reduction in cerebral blood flow. Because cerebral circulatory data were not available, subjects in the above study were classified on the basis of clinical and laboratory evidence of vascular disease anywhere in the circulatory system, including the heart, periphery, extracranial vessels, and brain. The lower graph in Figure 3 shows the relationship between the presence of such findings and blood pressure level. Among the control subjects, the incidence of vascular disease increased with blood pressure level in accordance with observations on cerebral atherosclerosis (Baker, Resch, and Loewenson 1969). The psychiatric patients, on the other hand, revealed a bimodal distribution, so that individuals at each end of the blood pressure continuum had a high incidence of clinically detectable vascular disease. It is the group with low blood pressure in the presence of vascular disease that was postulated to have cerebrovascular insufficiency. Interestingly, it was this group that showed the greatest prevalence of organic brain syndrome and diffuse EEG slowing, findings obtained in more than 70 percent of the cases.

In considering the role of vascular insufficiency, it should be noted that cerebral hemodynamic disturbances are not limited to intracranial vascular lesions, but may result from occlusion of the extracranial vessels as well (Adams, Smith, and Wylie 1963). Reduction in carotid artery diameter usually must exceed 50 percent before an appreciable drop in distal pressure occurs (Crawford et al. 1960). This agrees with the theoretical expectation that hemodynamics are not disturbed by a single stenosis, unless it is severe (May et al. 1963). On the other hand, milder multiple lesions and/or lumen narrowing over long sections of the vasculature might well produce significant blood pressure gradients (May, De Weese, and Rob 1963). The fact that there is a poor correlation between dementia and carotid or vertebral stenosis (Bryant et al. 1965; Kapp, Cook, and Paulson 1966) does not rule out the potential contribution of extracranial lesions when these are added to pathology elsewhere in the cardiovascular system, particularly in the contralateral vessels, circle of Willis, and collateral circulation (Fisher 1954). A precise understanding of the effect of vascular disease on cerebral blood flow in a given patient would require knowledge of pressure-flow relationships throughout the vascular tree.

The association of diffuse EEG slowing with low blood pressure in aged psychiatric patients suggests that blood pressure may directly influence cerebral blood flow and electrical activity. EEG slowing has been observed when blood pressure drops acutely in patients with carotid and basilar artery insufficiency (Meyer, Leiderman, and Denny-Brown 1956; Shanbrom and Levy 1957). Under normal conditions, however, mechanisms of autoregulation insure a remarkable stability of cerebral blood flow over a wide range of blood pressures (Harper 1966), so that a marked drop in pressure is necessary before blood flow is reduced. Since none of the patients in question had severe hypotension, it might be assumed either that lesser reductions in pressure were capable of producing cerebral ischemia, or that there was a loss of autoregulation resulting in a passive dependence of flow on pressure. There is indirect support for both of these possibilities. Finnerty, Witkin, and Fazekas (1954) observed that the decrease in blood pressure necessary to embarrass the cerebral circulation was less in patients who had hypertension and elevated cerebral vascular resistance; that is, blood flow reduction occurred at normotensive pressures. Furthermore, some patients with cerebrovascular disease showed impaired autoregulation (Agnoli et al. 1968; Paulson, Lassen, and Skinhøj 1970), a condition that may persist for days or weeks following an ischemic episode.

A clue concerning the relationship between cerebral blood flow and blood pressure in aged psychiatric patients is provided by Hedlund et al. (1964), who studied 16 patients with cerebral atherosclerosis, 5 of whom were demented. Figure 4 presents these findings,

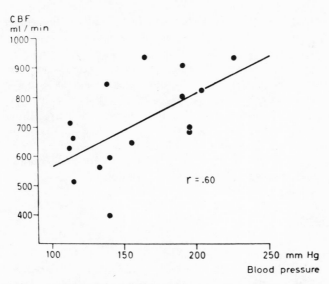

Figure 4. Cerebral blood flow (CBF) plotted as a function of systolic blood pressure in 16 patients, five of whom were demented, with clinical and/or radiological evidence of cerebrovascular disease. The correlation of +.60 is significant at the .02 level. From Hedlund et al. 1964.

which yielded a significant product-moment correlation of +.60 between the two variables. No correlation was found in patients with minimal evidence of vascular disease. Since the relationship was across individuals, rather than within individuals, it is not possible to infer impairment of autoregulation. Nevertheless, these findings do suggest a dependence of blood flow on blood pressure that is consistent with the EEG results described above.

More direct evidence for a relationship between cerebral blood flow and EEG in organic brain syndrome is provided by Obrist et al. (1963), who also studied oxygen uptake. Table 1 presents correlation coefficients between two EEG variables and cerebral vascular resistance (CVR), cerebral blood flow (CBF), and cerebral metabolic rate for

TABLE 1
Product-Moment Correlations between Cerebral Circulatory Variables
and EEG in Two Groups of Elderly Subjects

	Healthy Controls		Organic Brain Syndrome	
	Peak EEG Freq. (N = 24)	% - Slow Activity (N = 27)	Peak EEG Freq. (N = 17)	% - Slow Activity (N = 20)
CVR	+.02	- .07	- .48	+.52*
CBF	+.02	- .01	+.47	- .57*
CMRO$_2$	.00	+ .14	+.74**	- .78**

* Significant at the .05 level.
** Significant at the .001 level.

oxygen ($CMRO_2$), both in demented elderly patients and healthy controls. Peak EEG frequency refers to the modal point of the frequency spectrum, which primarily reflects the dominant rhythm; %-slow activity indicates the proportion of time waves below 7 cps appeared in the tracing. Whereas there was little or no correlation between EEG and any of the circulatory variables in the healthy old subjects, several significant coefficients were obtained in the patient group. The signs indicate that increased EEG slowing was associated with greater circulatory impairment, a finding recently confirmed in demented patients by Ingvar and Gustafson (1970). The fact that the highest correlations in Table 1 were with oxygen uptake is consistent with the known effects of cerebral hypoxia on EEG frequency (Gastaut and Meyer 1961). Whether such findings can be explained on the basis of hypoxia, however, depends on the relationship between hemodynamic and metabolic variables discussed below.

Cerebral Hemodynamic and Metabolic Variables

In 1956, Kety reviewed the available cerebral blood flow literature on neurologically normal subjects ranging from childhood to senescence. When plotted against age, both CBF and $CMRO_2$ revealed a small but nevertheless progressive decline in later life that paralleled the decrease reported for cortical neuron density (Brody 1955). Kety proposed two alternative hypotheses to explain the concomitant age-related decline in cerebral blood flow and metabolism: (1) that circulatory impairment results in reduced metabolic activity, and (2) that decreased metabolism results in reduced blood flow. The first hypothesis is consistent with the high incidence of vascular disease in senescence, a condition that might limit cerebral oxygen delivery, while the second is consistent with the capacity of the cerebral circulation to adjust to the lesser metabolic and functional demands of the aging brain. Since blood flow reduction might be attributed to either or both of these mechanisms, it becomes difficult to interpret the significance of a given measurement. This is particularly troublesome in patients with dementia, where it is desirable to distinguish blood flow reductions that are the direct result of vascular disease from those that are secondary to neuronal degeneration (O'Brien and Mallett 1970).

A possible way of assessing the contribution of vascular disease to cerebral blood flow changes is to determine the reactivity of the vasculature to altered CO_2 concentrations. Although carbon dioxide is one of the most potent cerebral vasodilators, many patients with vascular disease fail to show the expected increase in cerebral blood flow following CO_2 inhalation, an impairment that may be either regional or generalized (Fieschi et al. 1969). Some years ago, Novack et al.(1953) proposed that inhalation of 5-percent CO_2 might help to identify individuals with high cerebral vascular resistance due to arteriosclerosis, since in their experience such patients usually showed reduced blood flow responses. Schieve and Wilson (1953) went a step further and suggested that blood flow responses to CO_2 might help to differentiate dementias with a vascular etiology from those caused by primary parenchymal degeneration. According to their data, cerebral vessels react normally in the latter condition. Unfortunately, this hypothesis has never been adequately tested, no doubt because of the difficulty of justifying invasive blood flow techniques in both demented patients and elderly control subjects. The recent development of a noninvasive method for estimating cerebral blood flow, based on xenon[133] inhalation (Obrist et al. 1967), safely permits the multiple procedures required to explore this possibility. Preliminary studies have shown that the xenon inhalation method is quite sensitive to age changes and to variations in arterial pCO_2 (Obrist et al. 1971).

The newer radioisotopic methods for determining regional cerebral blood flow permit a further extension and refinement of hemodynamic studies on aging and mental deterioration. Obrist et al. (1970) observed that 5 of 10 elderly patients with organic brain syndrome had focal blood flow reductions confined to the anterior temporal-inferior frontal region. The predilection of this region for blood flow reduction in dementia has been confirmed by Ingvar and Gustafson (1970) and by Simard et al. (1971). Regional cerebral blood flow methods can also provide information on the relative tissue weights of grey and white matter, which vary in relation to the extent of cerebral atrophy (Høedt-Rasmussen and Skinhøj 1966) and the severity of intellectual deterioration (Obrist et al. 1970). These studies are merely suggestive; certainly, much more research is needed on both regional blood flow patterns and relative tissue weights as they relate to normal aging and to intellectual impairment. The noninvasive inhalation method described above, which is also regional, should facilitate such investigations.

Perhaps the most promising area for future study is the interrelation of hemodynamic and metabolic variables. In his discussion of aging, Kety (1956) argued that information about arteriovenous oxygen differences might shed light on cerebral blood flow alterations in senescence. The arteriovenous oxygen difference $[(A-V)O_2]$ can be expressed as a ratio between the oxygen utilization of a tissue and its blood flow, thus serving to indicate the adequacy of the circulation (Kety et al. 1950). Rearrangement of the Fick equation for oxygen uptake by the brain yields: $CMRO_2/CBF = (A-V)O_2$, where the A-V difference is expressed in cc of O_2 per 100 ml of blood obtained from arterial and jugular venous samples. When CBF decreases in response to a fall in $CMRO_2$ (as in anesthesia and certain types of coma), $(A-V)O_2$ is essentially unchanged, indicating an adjustment of blood flow to the lesser metabolic demands of the tissue. However, when CBF declines because of ischemia, the A-V difference increases, indicating that the brain is extracting more oxygen per unit of blood. Up to a point, a widened A-V difference can compensate for a reduction in blood flow, thereby maintaining a stable $CMRO_2$. The circulatory insufficiency in this case is merely relative. Failure of the compensatory mechanism occurs, however, when venous pO_2 reaches a lower limit (about 20 mm Hg), thus forcing $CMRO_2$ to decline. Here, a true circulatory insufficiency exists with resulting tissue hypoxia. Even when $CMRO_2$ is not depressed, a widened A-V difference can serve as a clue to impending or incipient cerebral hypoxia, the threshold of which may be crossed during minor hemodynamic disturbances. In cerebrovascular disease, inhomogeneous perfusion may result in some brain regions being affected earlier and to a greater degree than others.

A series of studies carried out at the National Institutes of Health (Dastur et al. 1963) offers some insight into $(A-V)O_2$ changes associated with normal aging, vascular disease, and dementia. Table 2 summarizes these findings. Whereas CBF, $(A-V)O_2$, and $CMRO_2$ were essentially the same in the normal young and elderly groups, subjects with mild, asymptomatic vascular disease showed a significant reduction in CBF that was associated with a rise in $(A-V)O_2$. Since the two variables tended to offset each other, $CMRO_2$ was unchanged. In the case of organic brain syndrome, the decline in CBF was not associated with an increase in $(A-V)O_2$, but rather was correlated with a reduction in $CMRO_2$. Sokoloff (1966) interpreted these results to indicate that, in the early stages of vascular disease, reductions in cerebral blood flow are the result of circulatory insufficiency, while in the later stages of the disease process (after tissue damage has occurred), reduced blood flow is secondary to a depression of the cerebral metabolic rate. Since asymptomatic vascular disease was associated with mild cognitive impairment, he further argued that circulatory disturbances may serve as a pacemaker for age changes in the brain.

The above findings are consistent with previous investigations by Scheinberg (1950a) and by Heyman et al. (1953) on patients with cerebrovascular disease. In these studies, reduced CBF and widened A-V oxygen differences were observed following acute cerebrovascular episodes, usually with only minimal alterations in $CMRO_2$. However, in cases with long-standing cerebrovascular disease, particularly those with progressive mental deterioration, the A-V differences were not as great, and cerebral blood flow

TABLE 2

Relation of Cerebral Circulatory and Metabolic Variables to Aging, Vascular Disease, and Mental Status†

	No. Cases	Mean Age	CBF (ml/100gm/min)	$(A-V)O_2$ (vol.%)	$CMRO_2$ (cc/100gm/min)
From Dastur et al. 1963					
Young controls	15	21	62.1 ±2.9	5.70 ±.30	3.51 ±.21
Normal Elderly	26	71	57.9 ±2.1	5.88 ±.17	3.33 ±.08
Asymptomatic vascular disease	15	73	50.8* ±2.7	6.79* ±.45	3.34 ±.14
Organic brain syndrome	10	72	48.5* ±3.8	5.69 ±.23	2.72* ±.18

† Means and standard errors are shown for the physiologic data.
* Significantly different from young controls ($p < .05$).

tended to parallel decreases in oxygen uptake. Further recent confirmation of these findings is provided by Géraud et al. (1969), who studied three groups of patients with vascular disease of different severity. When compared with normal controls and patients with no cerebral manifestations, subjects who had clinically evident cerebral ischemia showed increased A-V differences. Mentally deteriorated patients, on the other hand, revealed normal or slightly reduced $(A-V)O_2$.

The several studies cited above lend support to the notion that increased arteriovenous oxygen differences occur during the early ischemic stages of a circulatory disorder, and that $(A-V)O_2$ is essentially normal in the later stages after cerebral degenerative changes have occurred. As a supplement to cerebral blood flow measurements, $(A-V)O_2$ determinations would seem capable of differentiating blood flow reductions due to circulatory impairment from those that result from a depressed cerebral metabolism. In patients with declining intellectual function, such a distinction is of considerable importance, since it may have relevance to the etiology of the disorder. Dementias due to primary parenchymal degeneration might be expected to show little or no increase in $(A-V)O_2$, as in cases of brain atrophy (Lassen, Munck, and Tottey 1957) and Wernicke-Korsakoff syndrome (Shimojyo, Scheinberg, and Reinmuth 1967). Dementias secondary to cerebrovascular insufficiency, on the other hand, particularly in the early stages, might be expected to show significant increases in $(A-V)O_2$. Further carefully controlled studies are needed to assess the extent to which this variable may be of value in clinical research.

Oxygen uptake is only one aspect of cerebral metabolic function deserving study in the aged brain. As might be expected, glucose metabolism also undergoes changes with age and mental status (Dastur et al. 1963; Sokoloff 1966). More elaborate metabolic studies seem desirable, particularly an investigation of anaerobic glycolysis and its relationship to normal oxidative metabolism. Experimental studies on hypoxia in man have clearly shown increased lactic acid production and decreased oxygen-to-glucose ratios (Cohen et al. 1967). Since the shift to anaerobic glycolysis occurs early, long before oxygen supplies have been depleted, it could serve as a sensitive index of cerebral ischemia. Preliminary studies on carbohydrate metabolism in acute stroke patients have shown the expected increase in lactate production indicative of such a shift (Meyer et al. 1969).

From the above review, it is obvious that considerably more information is needed on cerebral hemodynamic and metabolic variables in relation to age and mental function. The various studies suggest that, given the continued development and refinement of techniques, investigations on the pathophysiology of circulatory disorders may provide some useful insight into aging processes in the brain.

References

Adams, J.E.; Smith, M.C.; and Wylie, E.J. 1963. Cerebral blood flow and hemodynamics in extracranial vascular disease: Effect of endarterectomy. *Surgery* 53:449.

Agnoli, A.; Fieschi, C.; Bozzao, L.; Battistini, N.; and Prencipe, M. 1968. Autoregulation of cerebral blood flow: Studies during drug-induced hypertension in normal subjects and in patients with cerebral vascular diseases. *Circulation* 38: 800.

Bailey, O.T. 1963. Influence of hypoxia in various diseases. In *Selective Vulnerability of the Brain in Hypoxaemia*. J.P. Schadé and W.H. McMenemey (eds.). Philadelphia: F.A. Davis, p. 227.

Baker, A.B.; Resch, J.A.; and Loewenson, R.B. 1969. Hypertension and cerebral atherosclerosis. *Circulation* 39:701.

Birren, J.E.; Botwinick, J.; Weiss, A.D.; and Morrison, D.F. 1963. Interrelations of mental and perceptual tests given to healthy elderly men. In *Human Aging: A Biological and Behavioral Study*. PHS Publication No. 986. Washington, D.C.: U.S. Govt. Printing Office, p. 143.

Brody, H. 1955. Organization of the cerebral cortex. III. A study of aging in the human cerebral cortex. *J. Comp. Neurol.* 102: 511.

Brody, H. 1970. Structural changes in the aging nervous system. *Interdiscipl. Topics Geront.* 7: 9.

Bryant, L.R.; Eiseman, B.; Spencer, F.C.; and Lieber, A. 1965. Frequency of extracranial cerebrovascular disease in patients with chronic psychosis. *New Eng. J. Med.* 272: 12.

Busse, E.W., and Wang, H.S. 1972. The multiple factors contributing to dementia in old age. In *Proceedings of the Fifth World Congress on Psychiatry*. Princeton, N.J.: Excerpta Medica (in press).

Cohen, P.J.; Alexander, S.C.; Smith, T.C.; Reivich, M.; and Wollman, H. 1967. Effects of hypoxia and normocarbia on cerebral blood flow and metabolism in conscious man. *J. Appl. Physiol.* 23: 183.

Corday, E.; Rothenberg, S.F.; and Putnam, T.J. 1953. Cerebral vascular insufficiency. *Arch. Neurol. Psychiat.* 69: 551.

Corsellis, J.A.N. 1962. *Mental Illness and the Ageing Brain*. London: Oxford University Press.

Crawford, E.S.; DeBakey, M.E.; Blaisdell, F.W.; Morris, G.C., Jr.; and Fields, W.S. 1960. Hemodynamic alterations in patients with cerebral arterial insufficiency before and after operation. *Surgery* 48: 76.

Dastur, D.K.; Lane, M.H.; Hansen, D.B.; Kety, S.S.; Butler, R.N.; Perlin, S.; and Sokoloff, L. 1963. Effects of aging on cerebral circulation and metabolism in man. In *Human Aging: A Biological and Behavioral Study*. PHS Publication No. 986. Washington, D.C.: U.S. Govt. Printing Office, p. 57.

Denny-Brown, D. 1960. Recurrent cerebrovascular episodes. *Arch. Neurol.* 2: 194.

Denny-Brown, D., and Meyer, J.S. 1957. The cerebral collateral circulation. 2. Production of cerebral infarction by ischemic anoxia and its reversibility in early stages. *Neurology* 7: 567.

Drake, W.E., Jr., and Drake, M.A.L. 1968. Clinical and angiographic correlates of cerebrovascular insufficiency. *Amer. J. Med.* 45: 253.

Eisdorfer, C. 1967. Psychologic reaction to cardiovascular change in the aged. *Mayo Clin. Proc.* 42: 620.

Eisenberg, S.; Madison, L.; and Sensenbach, W. 1960. Cerebral hemodynamic and metabolic studies in patients with congestive heart failure. *Circulation* 21: 704.

Ewalt, J.R., and Ruskin, A. 1944. The electroencephalogram in patients with heart disease. *Texas Rep. Biol. Med.* 2: 161.

Fazekas, J.F., and Alman, R.W. 1964. The role of hypotension in transitory focal cerebral ischemia. *Amer. J. Med. Sci.* 248: 567.

Fieschi, C.; Agnoli, A.; Prencipe, M.; Battistini, N.; Bozzao, L.; and Nardini, M. 1969. Impairment of the regional vasomotor response of cerebral vessels to hypercarbia in vascular diseases. *Europ. Neurol.* 2: 13.

Finnerty, F.A., Jr.; Witkin, L.; and Fazekas, J.F. 1954. Cerebral hemodynamics during cerebral ischemia induced by acute hypotension. *J. Clin. Invest.* 33: 1227.

Fisher, C.M. 1954. Occlusion of the carotid arteries. *Arch. Neurol. Psychiat.* 72: 187.

Fisher, C.M. 1968. Dementia in cerebral vascular disease. In *Cerebral Vascular Diseases*. J.F. Toole, R.G. Siekert, and J.P. Whisnant (eds.). New York: Grune & Stratton, p. 232.

Gastaut, H., and Meyer, J.S. (eds.) 1961. *Cerebral Anoxia and the Electroencephalogram*. Springfield, Ill.: Charles C Thomas.

Géraud, J.; Bes, A.; Delpla, M.; and Marc-Vergnes, J.P. 1969. Cerebral arteriovenous oxygen differences. Reappraisal of their significance for evaluation of brain function. In *Research on the Cerebral Circulation.* J.S. Meyer, H. Lechner, and O. Eichhorn (eds.). Springfield, Ill.: Charles C Thomas, p. 209.

Harper, A.M. 1966. Autoregulation of cerebral blood flow: Influence of the arterial blood pressure on the blood flow through the cerebral cortex. *J. Neurol. Neurosurg. Psychiat.* 29: 398.

Harvald, B. 1958. EEG in old age. *Acta Psychiat. Scand.* 33: 193.

Hedlund, S.; Köhler, V.; Nylin, G.; Olsson, R.; Regnström, O.; Rothström, E.; and Åström, K.E. 1964. Cerebral blood circulation in dementia. *Acta Psychiat. Scand.* 40: 77.

Heyman, A.; Patterson, J.L., Jr.; Duke, T.W.; and Battey, L.L. 1953. The cerebral circulation and metabolism in arteriosclerotic and hypertensive cerebrovascular disease. *New Eng. J. Med.* 249: 223.

Høedt-Rasmussen, K., and Skinhøj, E. 1966. In vivo measurements of the relative weights of gray and white matter in the human brain. *Neurology* 16: 515.

Ingvar, D.H., and Gustafson, L. 1970. Regional cerebral blood flow in organic dementia with early onset. *Acta Neurol. Scand.* 46 (suppl. 43): 42.

Jalavisto, E. 1964/65.. On the interdependence of circulatory-respiratory and neural-mental variables. *Gerontologia* 10: 31.

Kannel, W.B. 1971. Current status of the epidemiology of brain infarction associated with occlusive arterial disease. *Stroke* 2: 295.

Kapp, J.; Cook, W.; and Paulson, G. 1966. Chronic brain syndrome: Arteriographic study in elderly patients. *Geriatrics* 21: 174.

Kendell, R.E., and Marshall, J. 1963. Role of hypotension in the genesis of transient focal cerebral ischaemic attacks. *Brit. Med. J.* 2: 344.

Kety, S.S. 1956. Human cerebral blood flow and oxygen consumption as related to aging. *Res. Publ. Ass. Nerv. Ment. Dis.* 35: 31.

Kety, S.S.; King, B.D.; Horvath, S.M.; Jeffers, W.A.; and Hafkenschiel, J.H. 1950. The effects of an acute reduction in blood pressure by means of differential spinal sympathetic block on the cerebral circulation of hypertensive patients. *J. Clin. Invest.* 29: 402.

Kezdi, P.; Zaks, M.S.; Costello, H.J.; and Boshes, B. 1965. The impact of chronic circulatory impairment on functioning of central nervous system. *Ann. Intern. Med.* 62:67.

Lassen, N.A.; Munck, O.; and Tottey, E.R. 1957. Mental function and cerebral oxygen consumption in organic dementia. *Arch. Neurol. Psychiat.* 77: 126.

Malamud, N. 1965. A comparative study of the neuropathologic findings in senile psychoses and in "normal" senility. *J. Amer. Geriat. Soc.* 13: 113.

May, A.G.; De Weese, J.A.; and Rob, C.G. 1963. Hemodynamic effects of arterial stenosis. *Surgery* 53: 513.

May, A.G.; Van de Berg, L.; De Weese, J.A.; and Rob, C.G. 1963. Critical arterial stenosis. *Surgery* 54: 250.

Meier, M.J. 1970. Objective behavioral assessment in diagnosis and prediction: Presentation 14. In *Behavioral Change in Cerebrovascular Disease.* A.L. Benton (ed.). New York: Harper & Row, p. 119.

Meyer, J.S.; Leiderman, H.; and Denny-Brown, D. 1956. Electroencephalographic study of insufficiency of the basilar and carotid arteries in man. *Neurology* 6: 455.

Meyer, J.S.; Ryu, T.; Toyoda, M.; Shinohara, Y.; Wiederhold, I.; and Guiraud, B. 1969. Evidence for a Pasteur effect regulating cerebral oxygen and carbohydrate metabolism in man. *Neurology* 19: 954.

Millikan, C.H. 1965. The pathogenesis of transient focal cerebral ischemia. *Circulation* 32: 438.

Novack, P.; Shenkin, H.A.; Bortin, L.; Goluboff, B.; and Soffe, A.M. 1953. The effects of carbon dioxide inhalation upon the cerebral blood flow and cerebral oxygen consumption in vascular disease. *J. Clin. Invest.* 32: 696.

O'Brien, M.D., and Mallett, B.L. 1970. Cerebral cortex perfusion rates in dementia. *J. Neurol. Neurosurg. Psychiat.* 33: 497.

Obrist, W.D. 1972. Problems of aging. In *Handbook of Electroencephalography and Clinical Neurophysiology*, vol. 6. A. Rémond (ed.). Amsterdam: Elsevier Publ. Co. (in press).

Obrist, W.D., and Bissell, L.F. 1955. The electroencephalogram of aged patients with cardiac and cerebral vascular disease. *J. Geront.* 10: 315.

Obrist, W.D.; Busse, E.W.; Eisdorfer, C.; and Kleemeier, R.W. 1962. Relation of the electroencephalogram to intellectual function in senescence. *J. Geront.* 17: 197.

Obrist, W.D.; Busse, E.W.; and Henry, C.E. 1961. Relation of electroencephalogram to blood pressure in elderly persons. *Neurology* 11: 151.

Obrist, W.D.; Chivian, E.; Cronqvist, S.; and Ingvar, D.H. 1970. Regional cerebral blood flow in senile and presenile dementia. *Neurology* 20: 315.

Obrist, W.D.; Sokoloff, L.; Lassen, N.A.; Lane, M.H.; Butler, R.N.; and Feinberg, I. 1963. Relation of EEG to cerebral blood flow and metabolism in old age. *Electroenceph. Clin. Neurophysiol.* 15: 610.

Obrist, W.D.; Thompson, H.K.; King, C.H.; and Wang, H.S. 1967. Determination of regional cerebral blood flow by inhalation of 133-xenon. *Circ. Res.* 20: 124.

Obrist, W.D.; Thompson, H.K.; Wang, H.S.; and Cronqvist, S.A. 1971. A simplified procedure for determining fast compartment rCBFs by ^{133}xenon inhalation. In *Brain and Blood Flow*. R.W.R. Russell (ed.). London: Pitman Publ. Co., p. 11. i i

Paulson, O.B. 1971. Cerebral apoplexy (stroke): Pathogenesis, pathophysiology and therapy as illustrated by regional blood flow measurements in the brain. *Stroke* 2: 327.

Paulson, O.B.; Lassen, N.A.; and Skinhøj, E. 1970. Regional cerebral blood flow in apoplexy without arterial occlusion. *Neurology* 20: 125.

Reitan, R.M. 1970. Objective behavioral assessment in diagnosis and prediction: Presentation 15. In *Behavioral Change in Cerebrovascular Disease*. A.L. Benton (ed.). New York: Harper & Row, p. 155.

Riggs, H.E., and Wahal, K.M. 1962. Role of cardiovascular insufficiency in intellectual deterioration in senium. *Geriatrics* 17: 26.

Roth, M. 1971. Classification and aetiology in mental disorders of old age: Some recent developments. In *Recent Developments in Psychogeriatrics*. D.W.K. Kay and A. Walk (eds.). Ashford, U.K.: Headley Bros., p. 1.

Rothschild, D. 1942. Neuropathologic changes in arteriosclerotic psychoses and their psychiatric significance. *Arch. Neurol. Psychiat.* 48: 417.

Schadé, J.P., and McMenemey, W.H. (eds.) 1963. *Selective Vulnerability of the Brain in Hypoxaemia*. Philadelphia: F.A. Davis.

Scheinberg, P. 1950a. Cerebral blood flow in vascular disease of the brain. *Amer. J. Med.* 8: 139.

Scheinberg, P. 1950b. Cerebral circulation in heart failure. *Amer. J. Med.* 8: 148.

Schieve, J.F., and Wilson, W.P. 1953. The influence of age, anesthesia and cerebral arteriosclerosis on cerebral vascular activity to CO_2. *Amer. J. Med.* 15: 171.

Shanbrom, E., and Levy, L. 1957. The role of systemic blood pressure in cerebral circulation in carotid and basilar artery thromboses. *Amer. J. Med.* 23: 197.

Shapiro, W., and Chawla, N.P.S. 1969. Observations on the regulation of cerebral blood flow in complete heart block. *Circulation* 40: 863.

Shimojyo, S.; Scheinberg, P.; and Reinmuth, O. 1967. Cerebral blood flow and metabolism in the Wernicke-Korsakoff syndrome. *J. Clin. Invest.* 46: 849.

Simard, D.; Olesen, J.; Paulson, O.B.; Lassen, N.A.; and Skinhøj, E. 1971. Regional cerebral blood flow and its regulation in dementia. *Brain* 94: 273.

Simon, A., and Malamud, N. 1965. Comparison of clinical and neuropathological findings in geriatric mental illness. In *Psychiatric Disorders in the Aged*. Manchester, U.K.: Geigy Ltd., p. 322.

Sokoloff, L. 1961. Aspects of cerebral circulatory physiology of relevance to cerebrovascular disease. *Neurology* 11: 34.

Sokoloff, L. 1966. Cerebral circulatory and metabolic changes associated with aging. *Res. Publ. Ass. Nerv. Ment. Dis.* 41: 237.

Spieth, W. 1964. Cardiovascular health status, age, and psychological performance. *J. Geront.* 19: 277.

Sulg, I.A.; Cronqvist, S.; Schüller, H.; and Ingvar, D.H. 1969. The effect of intracardial pacemaker therapy on cerebral blood flow and electroencephalogram in patients with complete atrioventricular block. *Circulation* 39: 487.

Szafran, J. 1963. Age differences in choice reaction time and cardio-vascular status among pilots. *Nature* 200: 904.

Tomlinson, B.E.; Blessed, G.; and Roth, M. 1970. Observations on the brains of demented old people. *J. Neurol. Sci.* 11: 205.

Turton, E.C. 1958. The EEG as a diagnostic and prognostic aid in the differentiation of organic disorders in patients over 60. *J. Ment. Sci.* 104: 461.

Wilkie, F., and Eisdorfer, C. 1971. Intelligence and blood pressure in the aged. *Science* 172: 959.

Young, W.; Gofman, J.W.; Malamud, N.; Simon, A.; and Waters, E.S.G. 1956. The interrelationship between cerebral and coronary atherosclerosis. *Geriatrics* 11: 413.

Zülch, K.J. 1969. Reconsiderations of the clinical problem of cerebrovascular insufficiency. In *Research on the Cerebral Circulation.* J.S. Meyer, H. Lechner, and O. Eichhorn (eds.). Springfield, Ill.: Charles C Thomas, p. 1.

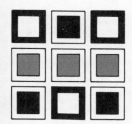

Laboratory Adjuncts to Differential Diagnosis

William S. Fields, M.D.

The University of Texas Medical School at Houston
Houston, Texas

This presentation should really be entitled "What can the laboratory contribute to the diagnosis and management of the illness of a person with clinical manifestations of an aging brain?"

Obviously, a title must be shorter, but by making it so it often becomes misleading. Those who have read the title and expect very much new information are doomed to dreadful disappointment. It may be equally important, however, to emphasize the futility and unwarranted expense of employing certain laboratory examinations in aged persons for practical purposes, although they do have some value as research tools.

Very few useful data have come from epidemiologic surveys on the incidence and prevalence of senile mental disorders. What we know has been obtained for the most part from studies of institutionalized individuals and provides only meager clues.

Dementia is a word many physicians are reluctant to use, even in this enlightened age. It still elicits a certain image and carries a certain social stigma for the patient and his family. Yet each year that we find the life expectancy of the average individual lengthening, there is a resultant increase in the number of elderly persons suffering from diminished intellectual capacity, or from intellectual incapacity.

Records and statistical reports obtained from acute and chronic hospitals and from nursing homes frequently indicate a diagnosis of "generalized" cerebral arteriosclerosis, or simply cerebral arteriosclerosis, as a substitute for the correct diagnosis of senile or presenile dementia. This is done sometimes out of kindness, which no one can fault, but it is more frequently the result of a widespread misconception among physicians that loss of intellectual function is a direct consequence of impaired cerebral circulation. The

135

problem is compounded by the fact that arteriosclerosis, or more specifically atherosclerosis, commonly occurs in the same age groups as senile and even presenile dementia. Another reason vascular disease may be implicated is that the physician is reluctant to place in the chart a diagnosis that might lead to the patient's exclusion from insurance coverage.

These factors have lead to the creation of a pathogenetic hypothesis of "arteriosclerotic dementia" that is highly questionable, to say the least, and difficult to support with clinical or laboratory evidence. There is no question that impairments of communication and of intellectual function can result from repeated small infarcts within the central nervous system, but invariably there is some associated evidence in such cases of other specific neurological deficits in motor or sensory function or both (Dupré and Devaux 1901; Ferrand 1902). Even in persons suffering from long-standing diabetes, particularly juvenile diabetes, in whom there is evidence of retinopathy, nephropathy, and other manifestations of arteriolopathy, one does not encounter encephalopathy that resembles the clinical picture of dementia unless there is evidence of cerebral malfunction in other spheres as well.

There is great difficulty in correlating the extent of clinical mental deficit with the degree of vascular change as observed by the pathologist. When both marked cortical atrophy and advanced atherosclerosis are observed in the same individual, one is tempted to ascribe one event to the other when they are more than likely coincidental. It is a well recognized fact that extensive and advanced atherosclerosis of the cerebral vessels may be present in persons whose intellectual capabilities are not noticeably impaired and, conversely, clinical evidence of advanced dementia may be unaccompanied by pathological changes in the vasculature. In other words, arteriosclerosis is basically a "non-cause" of senile dementia (Menken 1971).

There is a growing body of pathological evidence that senile dementia is not an entity *sui generis*, but merely Alzheimer's disease of later onset. If one is hesitant to use the term Alzheimer's disease as an acceptable description for both presenile dementia and dementia of later onset, it might be more acceptable to employ the longer but more descriptive term, namely, "primary cerebral neuronal degeneration."

Pneumoencephalography has long been used as a procedure for confirming the presence of cerebral atrophic change. It has been suggested that cortical atrophy in the presence of ventricles of normal or nearly normal size is compatible with primary neuronal degeneration, whereas ventricular enlargement with little or no evidence of cortical atrophy is most likely the result of vascular disease. Pathological studies, however, fail to confirm this suggested clinical-radiological correlation in the majority of cases. Pneumoencephalography, therefore, is a well accepted method of confirming one's clinical suspicion of a loss of cerebral tissue mass, but it cannot be considered helpful in providing clues with respect to the etiology.

It follows as a matter of natural course that if one adheres to the concept that the majority of mental impairments in the elderly is due to either cerebrovascular insufficiency or cerebral arteriosclerosis, then one ought to be able to make some determination with respect to diagnosis and therapy by utilizing laboratory tests that are available for *study of cerebral circulation*.

Reduction in both total and regional cerebral blood flow has been reported in dementia by a number of authors (Kety 1956; Lassen, Feinberg, and Lane 1960). More recently, O'Brien and Mallett (1970) tried to distinguish between primary neuronal degenerations and what they refer to as "secondary" dementia. In the latter category they place those persons in whom the implied etiology is of a vascular nature. They postulated that the cerebral blood flow in patients with primary neuronal degeneration might differ from that of patients whose dementia was secondary to vascular disease. In the first instance, the loss of neurons is the result of a cellular abnormality and the blood supply is unaffected. Cerebral blood flow, however, is very closely adjusted to the metabolic demand. Since the degenerative process in the brain primarily affects the more metabolically active cells and they are replaced by less metabolically active cells, some reduction in flow proportional to this reduced demand would be expected.

When dementia is secondary to vascular disease, healthy neurons are threatened by the inadequacy of the blood supply. One would anticipate, first, an increase in arteriovenous oxygen and glucose differences, and this phenomenon has been observed by several investigators. Cell death eventually occurs when this compensatory mechanism breaks down. Under the latter circumstances, the cerebral cortical perfusion rate is likely to be diminished early in the course of the disease, and the reduction would be expected to be disproportionate to the degree of mental impairment. This differentiation probably applies only early in the disease since long-standing cases of either type are likely to show atrophy due to reduced cell mass and reduced flow.

O'Brien and Mallett made a further attempt to correlate the degree of ventricular dilatation and the degree of cortical atrophy observed in a pneumoencephalogram with the cerebral blood flow. They postulated that, in patients who showed marked ventricular dilatation with a relatively intact cortex, these changes might have a vascular basis, whereas, in those with cortical atrophy and little or no ventricular enlargement, the changes might be based on primary neuronal degeneration. The investigators were unable, however, to substantiate this and found no correlation between the cerebral blood flow and the size of the ventricles or the degree of cortical atrophy.

Irrespective of the techniques used to measure cerebral cortical perfusion and cerebral blood flow, it is obviously important to compare both total and regional flow rates in elderly demented patients with those of a group of normal subjects matched for age. Unfortunately, this is not practicable with the methods for measuring cerebral blood flow available at the present time. Sokoloff (1966) found no significant change in cerebral blood flow with age alone, but his cases were highly selected and, consequently, his conclusions have been questioned by other investigators. Asymptomatic persons should be expected to show a fall in cerebral blood flow with age; this has been proved to be the case, and the decrease has been postulated to be due to subclinical vascular disease. Obviously, some degree of vascular change occurs in all persons of middle age or older, and progressive fallout of neurons can be expected from the adolescent period onward, with only the rate at which each occurs being variable. One would anticipate, therefore, a small progressive decrease in cortical perfusion rate with age in parallel with loss of the more metabolically active cells and, perhaps in addition, a variable loss due to the additive effect of degenerative vascular disease.

One may summarize the results of these studies by saying that patients with primary neuronal degeneration demonstrate a fall in cortical perfusion rate in relation to the loss of tissue and the decrease in metabolic demand. On the other hand, in patients whose dementia is secondary to vascular disease, the cortical perfusion rate is reduced early in the course of the disease, quite out of porportion to the degree of cortical atrophy demonstrated by a pneumoencephalographic study.

The *electroencephalogram* (EEG) is of limited value in a specific diagnosis in relation to the cause of aging. In persons who have diminished cardiac output or other reasons for cerebrovascular insufficiency, there is frequently increased theta activity, particularly in the temporal leads, and some slowing of the alpha rhythm. One may reasonably assume that these abnormalities have a circulatory basis since, in many patients, they will disappear after the administration of digitalis or the removal of obstructing arterial lesions. There is no correlation, however, between this type of change and loss of intellectual function.

Retrospective review of EEGs recorded in persons found later at postmortem examination to have had Alzheimer's disease shows a tendency to generalized slowing in all leads with a reduction in the amount of alpha activity. For these reasons, this test does not really contribute materially to an etiologic diagnosis and is useful only in elderly persons when there is some focal abnormality due to a specific identifiable pathological entity (Kellaway 1971).

Aortocranial arteriography has become a widely used radiological method for determining the pathological condition of the arteries and, when rapid serial films are taken, it may also provide useful information regarding total and regional flow and perfusion. New techniques using magnification may contribute more information about the condition of the intracranial circulation (Baker 1971).

Ten years ago, reconstructive surgery of extracranial arterial occlusive lesions became an important and accepted method for the relief of transient cerebral ischemic attacks and prevention of cerebral infarction. At that time, many vascular surgeons unfamiliar with the pathogenetic mechanisms and pathological changes underlying cerebrovascular disease tended toward an unfounded and unwarranted enthusiasm for operating on surgically accessible lesions in order to restore impaired intellectual functions. Usually, no distinction was made between the deficits associated with slow or reduced cerebral perfusion and the more classical picture of Alzheimer's disease or primary neuronal degeneration. In the former, one might anticipate an excellent response and in the latter, none. Such prognoses have subsequently proved to be correct.

At the height of interest in this problem, I had the opportunity to examine and follow during their hospital stay more than one hundred patients with dementia, admitted primarily for aortocranial arteriographic evaluation to reveal extracranial arterial lesions that might be amenable to surgery. Of the first hundred patients studied, only two had lesions — significant or insignificant — in the extracranial arteries.

It was of interest to me that in both cases there were audible midcervical bruits and a history of recurrent attacks of transient cerebral ischemia appropriate to the lesions demonstrated arteriographically. As one might have expected, operation in these two cases resulted in cessation of the attacks but no improvement in intellectual function. The arteriograms in the remaining cases were remarkably free of lesions in either the extracranial or intracranial arteries.

There is, however, a specific disturbance in intellectual function that accompanies some cases of extracranial arterial occlusive disease in which the large arterial trunks originating in the aortic arch are either markedly narrowed by atherosclerosis or completely occluded as a result of superimposed thrombosis. In such cases, the disease process is sometimes limited to these vessels, but in others, it is accompanied by lesions at more distally located extracranial sites, particularly in the region of the common carotid artery bifurcation. Physical examination of such patients reveals absence of arterial pulsations in the neck and upper limbs on one or both sides, arterial bruits, and reduction of brachial arterial blood pressure.

Studies of total cerebral blood flow in these patients demonstrate a sharp reduction in velocity of flow and transit time. Four-vessel arteriographic studies confirm the clinical suspicion of an occlusive process, and serial films will provide information regarding the rate of flow of the contrast material and the extent of compensatory collateral circulation. It is the latter which determines the extent of cerebral circulation and influences both the degree of functional impairment and the potentiality for restoration of function.

If the disease process is far enough advanced, and the compensatory circulation of borderline adequacy, then a specific clinical picture is produced. This has been referred to as the "low cerebral perfusion syndrome." It is characterized by general retardation of cerebration including inability to concentrate, inattention, and faulty judgment. Visual-motor and visual-perceptual impairments are common and can be readily demonstrated by the appropriate neuropsychological tests. The patient is usually aware of his problem to some extent, and his frustration and anxiety are thereby increased.

This state is reversible in most cases of this nature and the improvement in mental function consequent to surgical intervention is often dramatic. It is almost immediately apparent to the family, to business associates, to the physician, and to the patient himself. The change is not merely a qualitative one or an impression, but one that can be documented in most instances by markedly improved test performance. The change is obviously real enough and not related to a learning factor in the administration of the tests.

The following illustrates very well the clinical manifestations associated with this syndrome:

Mr. G.K., a 61-year-old general counsel for a large steel company in Ohio, was noted by his secretary and other business associates to be having great difficulty in handling his affairs during a period of five months prior to his admission to hospital. His secretary first noted that, even in the midst of his dictation which she took in shorthand, he would lose his train of thought and have great difficulty in recalling the subject material at hand. At first, she could read back to him the preceding sentence and he would be able to pick up where he left off. However, over a period of four or five weeks, he became increasingly inattentive and, on occasion, could not even finish a letter he had started. He was required to meet with other executives frequently in conference and this became increasingly difficult for him because of poor concentration and a shorter and shorter span of attention. He was aware of much of this difficulty himself, which created an even greater problem for him. The company went along for several months in the hope that he would improve and be able to carry on, but after he made several serious errors in judgment, they suggested that he take an early medical retirement.

The patient was sent to a company physician for evaluation. The physician could not obtain the right radial pulse, and when he took the blood pressure in each arm it was 40 mm lower on the right than on the left. He also noted that there were no pulsations over the carotid arteries on either side of the neck. He therefore recommended that the patient go elsewhere for further examination before making any decision regarding his future. There was no additional pertinent clinical history and the patient denied any visual, auditory, or vestibular symptoms. The only other clinical finding not previously recorded was a loud systolic bruit audible in the left supraclavicular region. Examination of the ocular fundi showed slowing of the circulation through the retinal arterioles.

A thoracic aortogram was done by retrograde femoral catheterization (Figure 1). This study revealed complete occlusion of the brachiocephalic trunk and left common carotid artery and 60 percent stenosis in the proximal portion of the left subclavian artery. Late films in the series showed filling of the distal neck vessels through collaterals with a 70 percent narrowing of the left internal carotid at its origin and minimal stenosis in the distal portion of the right common carotid. The intracranial vessels were not adequately visualized by this technique.

Two days later, a bypass graft was placed from the ascending aorta through the thoracic outlet to the left common carotid bifurcation, at which level an endarterectomy was performed. Extrathoracic side branches were placed from the main graft to each subclavian artery distal to the origin of the vertebral arteries.

The patient complained of severe headache for about 36 hours after surgery, but there was a remarkable and dramatic change in his mental capability. This continued to improve during the remainder of his hospital stay.

When he returned to Ohio, it was immediately apparent to the referring physician, his family, and his business associates that his intellectual capacity was restored to what it had been several years earlier. When seen again on a follow-up visit ten months after surgery, the improvement had obviously been maintained, the patient was working regularly, and his general outlook was considerably brighter.

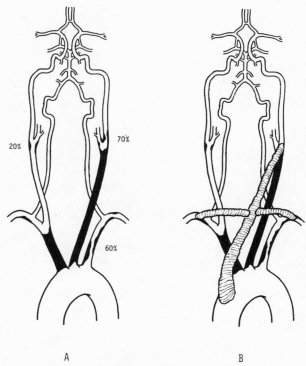

A   B

Figure 1. A. Location of lesions observed in preoperative arteriogram.
B. Diagram showing location of synthetic prosthetic bypass graft.

Unfortunately, persons with this type of vascular abnormality constitute only an exceedingly small percentage of the population affected by atherosclerosis involving the aortocranial arteries. Extracranial arterial lesions are at least twenty times more common at the level of the common carotid bifurcation and also more common and widespread in the intracranial branches. The clinical manifestations of lesions in these other locations are quite separate and distinct and are generally categorized as "transient cerebral ischemic attacks" or "completed stroke." Changes within the brain are secondary to thromboembolism in a high percentage of cases and to hemodynamic alterations of pressure and flow associated with inadequate circulation in others.

Cerebrospinal fluid examination has not been helpful in diagnosis of dementia. The fluid has been uniformly normal in autopsy-proved cases of Alzheimer's disease. In cases with cerebral arteriosclerosis, the fluid is also usually normal unless there is some complication, such as cerebral infarction, hemorrhage, uremia, or congestive heart failure.

One may find a protein content of greater than 40 mg per 100 cc in only an occasional uncomplicated case, but this of itself is not diagnostic (Merritt and Fremont-Smith 1938).

Since the diagnosis of Alzheimer's disease can be definitely established only by the pathologist, the question must be raised regarding the potentialities of *cerebral biopsy* in so-called degenerative disorders.

Several years ago, at another conference held in Houston, Dr. Robert Terry, a participant in this one, presented a very carefully considered and elegant paper on cerebral biopsy (Terry 1966). What he said then is as current today, particularly his comment that, "Since at present most of these diseases cannot be effectively treated, there is a serious moral problem involved in justifying cerebral biopsy."

If an autopsy will eventually be available, why should one even consider biopsy? Many enzymes quickly become inactive after death, and the ultrastructure of the brain undergoes very rapid alteration. The postmortem deterioration of the brain is even more rapid than in other organs and, therefore, if one wishes to prepare a specimen for electron microscopy, a biopsy is obviously required in order to provide an accurate demonstration of the *in vivo* enzymatic activity and ultrastructure.

Since no effective treatment can be offered these persons, it is imperative to review with the family the research nature of the procedure. Two additional considerations are also of the utmost importance: first, that the biopsy be postponed until late in the course of the progressive disorder and, second, that the procedure be undertaken only by a sufficiently well-equipped research team who are capable of properly removing and preparing with utmost care a specimen for study, so that the maximum amount of information can be obtained and correlated with the clinical data.

It should be evident from the foregoing that the laboratory has only a limited capability of providing information of diagnostic value during the life of the patient and even fewer data that will lead to effective therapeutic measures. The only exception of which I am aware and which I previously described is that of patients in whom there is a mental impairment clearly "secondary" to reduced cerebral cortical perfusion and a state of reversible malfunction of the neurons.

I trust that this rather nihilistic view of the value of laboratory procedures in the identification and understanding of the processes associated with aging will not long prevail.

References

Baker, H.L., Jr. 1971. Clinical usefulness of magnification cerebral angiography. *Radiology* 98:587.
Dupre, E., and Devaux, A. 1901. Foyers lacunaires de désintégration cérébrale (note sur le processus histogenique). *Rev. Neurol.* 9:653.
Ferrand, J. 1902. Essai sur l'hemiplegie des vieillards. Les lacunes de désintégration cérébrale. Paris Thesis.

Kellaway, P. 1971. Personal communication.

Kety, S.S. 1956. Human cerebral blood flow and oxygen consumption as related to ageing. *Ass. Res. Nerv. Ment. Dis. Proc.* 35:31.

Lassen, N.A.; Feinberg, I.; and Lane, M.H. 1960. Bilateral studies of cerebral oxygen uptake in the young and aged normal subjects and in patients with organic dementia. *J. Clin. Invest.* 39:491.

Menken, M. 1971. Cerebral arterial sclerosis: A non-cause of dementia. *J. Med. Soc. N.J.* 68:219.

Merritt, H.H., and Fremont-Smith, F. 1938. *The Cerebrospinal Fluid.* Philadelphia: Saunders.

O'Brien, M.D., and Mallett, B.L. 1970. Cerebral cortex perfusion rates in dementia. *J. Neurol. Neurosurg. Psychiat.* 33:497.

Sokoloff, L. 1966. Cerebral circulatory and metabolic changes associated with ageing. *Ass. Res. Nerv. Ment. Dis. Proc.* 41:237.

Terry, R.D. 1966. The value of cerebral biopsy. In *Neurological Diagnostic Techniques.* W.S. Fields (ed.). Springfield: Thomas.

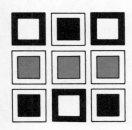

Autonomic Changes in Aging

Carl Eisdorfer, Ph.D., M.D.

Duke University Medical Center
Durham, North Carolina

The subject of my paper, reflecting as it does very different anatomic sites from the lofty location of the cortical complex, places me in an awkward position. It is hardly a case of bringing coals to Newcastle, but rather more analogous to delivering a bikini to a Bedouin tribesman. Not only is there a risk that it won't cover much but, besides, who needs it.

Introduction

Descartes has been translated (1892) to state, "there is a vast difference between mind and body, in respect that body, from its nature, is always divisible, and that mind is entirely indivisible." This orientation was elaborated and subsequently developed into the belief of a mind/body dualism which in turn has had a rather profound influence on the evolution of human biologic science including psychobiology, conceptually separating as it does the brain from the rest of the organism.

As we all know, advances in science are slow and laborious. It is not always easy to reject some concepts from our thinking, even after we reject their empirical validity, so I won't belabor any further this attempt to shake Cartesian dualism. Suffice it to say that my focus is upon the autonomic influences on behavior which, of course, interact with and must be mediated by the CNS.

The approach in this paper is an outgrowth of work undertaken several years ago in an area presumed to be related exclusively to central nervous system functioning but the work, as you will see, took a somewhat different turn.

Background

Something over a decade ago, I entertained the notion that in the central nervous system an active damping mechanism must be responsible for recovery from visual or auditory stimulation. This seemed to be the most appropriate way to explain the phenomenon of time lag between readiness for re-stimulation of young and old persons following an identical stimulus. Since the impression is that older persons are less subjectively stimulated by a given input than the young, it is difficult to explain why they take so much longer to recover to the point of being ready for re-stimulation. It was postulated that there is a decrement in some active neuronal process responsible for returning the information-processing capacity of aging persons to a resting level following stimulation. This, in turn, led to a number of studies of visual and kinesthetic aftereffects that I performed with my colleagues (Axelrod and Eisdorfer 1962 and 1964), and which also included a study of serial rote learning.

In the learning study (Eisdorfer, Axelrod, and Wilkie 1963), we demonstrated that comparable groups of old and young subjects showed significantly different patterns of improvement as we increased the rate of presentation of stimulus words in an eight-item serial rote learning paradigm. As the time limits were extended from 5 to 7 to 9 seconds between stimulus onset, younger subjects did not seem to profit very much. From 5 to 7 to 9 seconds, however, there was a significant monotonic change in the performance of our older subjects. An important consideration was that older subjects seemed to show improvement primarily as a function of an increased tendency to respond with increasing stimulus exposure time. It became quite clear after a number of experiments that the improvement in performance of aged persons on this learning task was, in fact, associated with more time to respond to the stimulus. We assumed that aging resulted in slowing of response speed even at this level, but experimental work also demonstrated, somewhat to our surprise, that it was not that older subjects could not respond under our most rapid pacing condition, but rather that they would not respond.

In an effort to establish the basis of this failure to respond and to view the effects of the learning challenge, we began to study the learning pattern simultaneously with free fatty acid mobilization. We chose free fatty acid because of the questionable reliability of serum catecholamine determination on small samples of blood, because urinary catechols would not do for concurrent study with the learning, and also because the galvanic skin response (GSR) changes in older persons were somewhat in the pale in my laboratory at that time due to our concern with the effects of skin changes with increasing age. Bloods were drawn using a Cournand needle or a catheter under local procaine anesthesia with the arm shielded from the subject; no pain was reported in these studies. It did appear that older persons demonstrated a pattern of free fatty acid mobilization significantly different from that of the young, and they reflected heightened and more persistent levels of autonomic activity than did our younger subjects. Both young and old showed parallel drops in mobilization levels for 30 minutes of the resting stage following insertion of the needle. The young peaked with the onset of learning, continued to show high levels for the two additional learning samples, and dropped off during the postlearning periods. Older persons showed curves that peaked 15 minutes after learning and stayed high for the remaining 45 minutes (Powell, Eisdorfer, and Bogdonoff 1964).

A study of mobilization of free fatty acids and of disappearance of isotopically labeled free fatty acids demonstrated that the differences we saw in our learning experiment were not simple functions of differences in the metabolism of older versus younger persons (Eisdorfer, Powell, Silverman, and Bogdonoff 1965). The apparent higher elevation and persistence of free fatty acid mobilization in older persons during the stress of the learning experiment led us to believe that perhaps much of the existing literature concerning depressed autonomic nervous system functioning in the aged was erroneous, or that using the same time sequence for old and young subjects might give an incomplete story. Moreover, Cohen and Shmavonian (1967) demonstrated heightened urinary catechol response to adrenalin in younger persons at 90 minutes, but they ignored the fact that at 180 minutes postinjection the response level of the young dropped below that of the aged subjects, whose responses still reflected a monotonic increase at the end of the three-hour study.

A word now about measures of autonomic nervous system arousal in older persons. While the psychophysiological literature has more than its share of studies of autonomic nervous system activity, a review of that literature reveals only a limited number of studies dealing with the aged. An excellent treatment of this subject is provided by Drs. Larry Thompson and Gail Marsh, who have completed a review of psychophysiologic studies of the aging for the forthcoming volume published by the American Psychological Association Task Force on Aging (Thompson and Marsh, in press). Botwinick and Kornetsky (1959 and 1960) used GSR in a conditioning study and found that autonomic reactivity was considerably less in their older than in their younger subjects. Shmavonian (1965) performed an autonomic conditioning experiment using the GSR coupled with plethysmography and EEG measures. He reported that the magnitude of conditioning of GSR responses was substantially less for old than for young individuals, and that vasomotor reactivity as measured by a finger plethysmograph also appeared to be diminished for the old. In contrast, the EEG measures showed greater reactivity for the old than the young.

Recent work by Morris and Thompson (1969), Nowlin, Thompson, and Eisdorfer (in press), and Thompson and Nowlin (in press), who investigated the phenomenon reported by Lacey and Lacey (1967 and 1970) involving heart rate deceleration prior to an imperative stimulus and the acceleration subsequent to the stimulus, has shown that the magnitude of blood pressure and heart rate change was considerably less in old as contrasted with younger subjects. While older persons do show changes in peripheral autonomic nervous system end organs — in that there is clear cardiovascular responsivity in relation to level of attention in the reaction-time situation — it is also apparent that the amplitude of change in the elderly is less than in the young.

Returning to our learning studies, one may recall that during learning, the aged were characterized by apparently heightened arousal patterns involving free fatty acid mobilization. The activation curve used by Malmo and a good many others holds that the relationship between performance and arousal (in this case, autonomic nervous system arousal) can be depicted by an inverted U-shaped curve. We hypothesized that aged subjects traditionally believed to be at the low end of the performance ordinate and activation abscissa might actually be functioning as if they were at the heightened end of the arousal dimension. It would follow, therefore, that a reduction in autonomic nervous system arousal in older persons would result in improved levels of performance. We seemed to substantiate this position in a study in which the task was made easier at the faster pace of learning by bringing in brighter subjects. Performance improved at the faster learning speeds and changes in the patterns of omission errors were as predicted (Eisdorfer and Service 1967). More important, however, it also followed that if we could modify ANS activity by direct action we ought to achieve the same effect.

In a recent study with Nowlin and Wilkie (Eisdorfer, Nowlin, and Wilkie 1970), we postulated that if performance in learning was being mediated by heightened ANS end organ activity, apparent learning should improve significantly with successful blockage of the effects of heightened autonomic nervous system arousal by a beta-adrenergic blocking agent. The hypothesis was tested by administering either 10 mg of propranolol or of saline solution intravenously shortly before subjects were given the learning task to perform. The results were quite striking. Not only was there a significant placebo effect, but there was a significant drug effect beyond the placebo effect. It was quite clear also that the drug did block free fatty acid mobilization for most of the study period and it also reduced and stabilized heart rate. It is interesting that, while GSR was somewhat more stable in the experimental group, this difference did not persist for the two-hour duration of the experiment. At this point, we were ready to accept that there was evidence for heightened ANS activity being associated with a deficit in learning performance and responsivity in older men, or at least that reduction in aspects of autonomic and organ activation was a significant variable. The mechanisms of greater interest perhaps lie in the CNS mediation of autonomic arousal and performance.

Discussion

The discrepancy between our data on free fatty acid mobilization and Shmavonian's EEG data and other findings on autonomic nervous system activity suggests three general themes which I would like to propose.

The first is that someone's data are wrong. Obviously, while I entertain this idea about my own work from time to time, it usually occurs to me at 2:00 or 2:30 a.m. while trying to get to bed after a rough day, and I muster all my psychodynamic and psychoanalytic background to suppress such ideas. The sorts of things I share with myself include the knowledge that our learning data have been replicated in our own laboratory many times, and, perhaps more important, that the general pattern of what we have described has been repeated in at least four or five other laboratories. The simultaneous autonomic measurements, however, are a little more complicated and no one has attempted to replicate them. Autonomic nervous system measures are subject to a variety of difficulties, and more information needs to be generated on these measures, vis à vis aging. As was pointed out earlier, the data provided by many studies are too limited in time to allow accurate conclusions. This is a specific age-related problem since short-term measurements of older people, who may mobilize more slowly, would not accurately assess the eventual peak level of activation. (In fact, in our laboratory the significant findings were clearest with learning.)

If we assume, however, that all the data are accurate, alternative interpretations suggest themselves. Thompson and Marsh (in press) have suggested that in the elderly human being, traditional autonomic measures may no longer adequately reflect the extent of autonomic nervous system arousal. We should bear in mind that different end organs controlled by the autonomic system may show quite different age effects, and this divergence may well occur with increasing frequency as age progresses. Thompson and Marsh also speculate that, since stimulation of the sympathetic and parasympathetic nervous systems is an important factor in free fatty acid mobilization, autonomic nervous system arousal might be interpreted as reflecting heightened stress when free fatty acid mobilization is high. This is, of course, substantiated by an extensive literature. They further suggest that perhaps the depressed level of GSR and cardiovascular responsivity, measured peripherally, is due to deterioration in the flexibility of those end organs. Certainly the cardiovascular system and the skin are notoriously susceptible to age effects. If Thompson and Marsh's explanation is correct, it is conceivable that there is heightened central nervous system activity in response to autonomic state; however, depending on the particular end organ being studied, the patterning might be quite different. It would suggest that a variety of consequences could be postulated if we assumed that some end organs were unable to function optimally and might be sending distorted messages back to the central nervous system. As a consequence, feedback from CNS to the periphery would be distorted to such an extent that the more sensitive end organs would be disproportionately activated and send back the signals of hyperarousal, thus shutting off CNS messages and creating eccentric CNS-ANS patterning. Given this system, behavioral effects might well involve withdrawal and inhibition.

It could be argued from such a model that despite heightened levels of serum catecholamines, the effect of a beta-blocking agent would be to diminish end organ arousal, resulting in the delivery of messages to the CNS that reflect this lowered end organ activity. In turn, this could increase the arousal pattern of the CNS. Clearly, joint ANS-CNS studies are required to investigate this possibility, and we are indeed initiating such studies at this time.

Advancing the hypothesis that aging has the result of producing unequal changes in regulatory processes at several levels of the organism, Frolkis (1965) and his colleagues at Kiev have accumulated an extensive array of data indicating changes in various parts of the neurohumoral regulatory system during aging. Using atropine and dihydroergotamine to block parasympathetic and sympathetic effects on the heart, Frolkis found a decrease in both sympathetic and parasympathetic influences on resting heart rate of aged rats. On the other hand, he also demonstrated that the same end organ, the heart, is more sensitive to direct action of the transmitter substance itself. In a variety of studies, he develops the same general theme by showing that small amounts of neurotransmitter applied directly to a target organ would have the same effect in the aged animal as in the young. His models included the nictitating membrane in cats' skeletal muscles sensitive to acetylcholine and the excitation threshold of visceral efferent nerves to electrical stimulation. In effect, Frolkis is saying that in aged persons the tissues seem to be less sensitive to neuronal influences but more sensitive to the neurotransmitter substance contained by those same nervous fibers. This probably is secondary to loss of neuronal tissue. What is being postulated is a new balance based upon a weakening of certain neuronal influences accompanied by increased sensitivity to neurohumoral factors, assuming that those humoral factors are present in diminished quantities.

Troyer (in press) interprets these findings to indicate that the aged person might be characterized by partial denervation hypersensitivity. Such hypersensitivity may occur when either acetylcholine- or noradrenaline-containing fibers are destroyed. As a result, the effector organ has a greater response to a given amount of its appropriate neurotransmitter. Frolkis does indeed show decreases in the tissue level of cholinesterase and acetylcholine associated with age. Troyer (in press) postulates a model of heightened threshold for end organ activity on the effector side. Impulses are harder to initiate and may travel a bit more slowly. On the afferent side, however, there may be greater sensitivity, particularly to heightened levels of activity in the case of the relatively intact end organ.

For the organism as a whole, many age-related observations are explainable as deficits in those aspects of behavior that require participation of sympathetic and parasympathetic activity. Frolkis's work showed that interoceptors seem to be substantially more sensitive in the aged than in the young. The pressure change necessary to elicit the pressor reflex from the carotid sinus in old animals was 50 percent smaller than that in the young. Indeed, this may go a long way toward explaining Thompson and Nowlin's findings of diminished cardiac rate and blood pressure changes with attention to a compelling stimulus. It may be that, in keeping with Lacey's hypothesis, this early inhibition with less cardiac deceleration in the aged produces the same amount of inhibition as occurs in the young. If we accept such a speculative model, the greater sensitivity of end organs to neurohumoral release in older persons may be viewed as possibly triggering a CNS deactivation which, in turn, would be reflected by impaired performance. Solid data on these issues would be very interesting. Perhaps what is important is the recognition that alterations in the autonomic nervous system which we do not fully appreciate may play an important role in explaining some of the central nervous system activity that is reflected in the behavior of aging persons. In the case of Eisdorfer and his colleagues, these alterations may help explain performance in learning;

in the case of Nowlin, Thompson, and his colleagues, they may be valuable in explaining cardiac patterning. On a gross level, they may well point to the greater sensitivity of older persons to internal somatic changes and, indeed, perhaps to behavior in the larger social context.

References

Axelrod, S., and Eisdorfer, C. 1962. Senescence and figural after-effects in two modalities. *J. Genet. Psychol.* 100:85.

Axelrod, S., and Eisdorfer, C. 1964. Senescence and figural after-effects in two modalities: A correlation. *J. Genet. Psychol.* 104:193.

Botwinick, J., and Kornetsky, C. 1959. Age differences in the frequency of the GSR during a conditioning experiment. *J. Geront.* 14:503.

Botwinick, J., and Kornetsky, C. 1960. Age differences in the acquisition and extinction of the GSR. *J. Geront.* 15:83.

Cohen, S.I., and Shmavonian, B.M. 1967. Catecholamines, vasomotor conditioning and aging. In *Endocrines and Aging.* L. Gitman (ed.). Springfield, Ill.: Charles C Thomas, p. 102.

Descartes, R. 1650 (trans. 1892). *Passions of the Soul.* Henry A.A. Torrey (trans.). New York: Henry Holt. pt. 1, p. 292. Original French, *Les passions de l'âme.* Amsterdam.

Eisdorfer, C.; Axelrod, S.; and Wilkie, F. 1963. Stimulus exposure time as a factor in serial learning in an aged population. *J. Abnorm. Soc. Psychol.* 67:594.

Eisdorfer, C.; Nowlin, J.B.; and Wilkie, F. 1970. Improvement of learning in the aged by modification of autonomic nervous system activity. *Science* 170:1327.

Eisdorfer, C.; Powell, A.H.; Silverman, G.; and Bogdonoff, M.D. 1965. The characteristics of lipid mobilization and peripheral disposition in aged individuals. *J. Geront.* 20:4.

Eisdorfer, C., and Service, C. 1967. Verbal rote learning and superior intelligence in the aged. *J. Geront.* 22:158.

Frolkis, V.V. 1965. Neuro-humoral regulations in the aging organism. *J. Geront.* 21(no. 2):161.

Lacey, J.I. 1967. Somatic response patterning and stress: Some revisions of activation theory. In *Psychological Stress: Issues in Research.* M.H. Appley and R. Trumball (eds.). New York: Appleton-Century-Crofts.

Lacey, J.I., and Lacey, B.C. 1970. Some autonomic-central nervous system interrelationships. In *Physiological Correlates of Emotion.* P. Black (ed.). New York: Academic Press, p. 205.

Morris, J.D., and Thompson, L.W. 1969. Heart rate changes in a reaction time experiment with young and aged subjects. *J. Geront.* 24 (no. 3):269.

Nowlin, J.B.; Thompson, L.W.; and Eisdorfer, C. in press. Cardiovascular response during reaction time performance. *Psychophysiology.*

Powell, A.H.; Eisdorfer, C.; and Bogdonoff, M.D. 1964. Physiologic response patterns observed in a learning task. *Arch. Gen. Psychiat.* 10:192.

Shmavonian, B.M.; Yarmat, A.J.; and Cohen, S.I. 1965. Relationships between autonomic nervous system and central nervous system in age differences in behavior. In *Behavior, Aging and the Nervous System.* A.T. Welford and J.E. Birren (eds.). Springfield, Ill.: Charles C Thomas, p. 235.

Thompson, L.W., and Marsh, G. in press. Psychophysiological studies of aging: Preliminary draft. American Psychological Assn. Task Force on Aging.

Thompson, L.W., and Nowlin, J.B. in press. Cortical slow potential and cardiovascular correlates of attention during reaction time performance. In *Intellectual Changes from Childhood through Maturity: Some Psychological and Biological Aspects.* L. Jarvik, C. Eisdorfer, and J. Blum (eds.). New York: Springer.

Troyer, W. in press. Mechanisms of brain body interaction in the aged. In *Intellectual Changes from Childhood through Maturity: Psychological and Biological Aspects.* L. Jarvik, C. Eisdorfer, and J. Blum (eds.). New York: Springer.

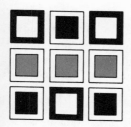

Differential Diagnosis of the Organic Mental Disorders in Elderly Patients

Joseph M. Foley, M.D.

School of Medicine, Case Western Reserve University, Cleveland, Ohio

Differential diagnosis of the behavioral disorders of the elderly must be made in the traditional pattern and with the traditional logic of medical diagnosis. It must not be solely or predominantly intuitive. It must not be prejudiced by a preconception that too much life lies behind and too little ahead. It must not be concerned exclusively with morbid anatomy.

The traditional sequence of effective diagnosis in medicine begins with an elicitation of the phenomena, the symptoms and signs of disease. These phenomena are then transformed into physiological context and the *physiological diagnosis* defines the nature of the disturbed function. The next step is the *anatomical diagnosis*, the identification of those areas which, when affected, produce this kind of physiological change. This level of diagnosis makes no presumptions about reversibility or irreversibility or about the nature of the lesion. The third step is *pathological diagnosis*, by which is meant both morbid anatomy and pathogenesis. Whereas the step from physiological to anatomical is reasonably simple and logical, the step from anatomical to pathological requires many sources of assistance from all the data available—system review, family history, the laboratory, the social situation, and the environment in which the phenomena arise. This last step is the one that requires all the skills of clinical medicine—the use of anatomy and physiology, the excursion into nonanatomical and nonphysiological details of the patient's life and circumstances, and of necessity, however regrettable, some of the educated guessing that is called intuition.

Differential diagnosis must be in these several hierarchies. It is necessary to know phenomenologically whether the patient is eccentric or delirious, physiologically whether his twitches are myoclonus or multiple tics, anatomically whether the cerebral cortex is diffusely involved or whether one temporal lobe is focally involved, and pathologically whether he has a meningioma or Alzheimer's disease. Some of the worst mistakes in diagnostic medicine result when a jump is made from phenomenology to pathology without the intermediate analysis of physiology and anatomy.

Applying this method to the differential diagnosis of the behavioral changes of old age is necessary if these disorders are to be given appropriate prognosis and management in any individual patient.

Prognosis and management must also be thought of in these categories. Misunderstandings about treatment objectives can be avoided if the physician knows clearly whether he is altering symptoms and signs, restoring disturbed physiology and anatomy, or altering or reversing the course of the underlying pathogenetic agent. This approach also reveals avenues of investigation that must be traveled before we can hope for a scientific understanding of the totality of this large problem.

The phenomena of disease are the symptoms and signs. In the behavioral disorders the phenomena are almost unlimited because human behavior is extremely complex. The patient may be glad or mad, happy or sad, content or miserable, exalted or depressed, conscious or stuporous, alert or apathetic, appropriate or absurd, silly or solemn, bright or dull, or one or another of hundreds, perhaps thousands, of possible antonymic combinations. In organic disturbances of behavior it is necessary to identify certain categories of phenomena in the search for a physiological diagnosis. Among these would be disorientation, confusion, stupor, coma, depression, anxiety, inappropriateness, dementia, psychosis, and the like. Some of these terms have agreed-upon meaning, but some others need to be defined because there has been no unanimity about how to use them.

Disorientation is an inability to make true identification of persons, places, times, things, and their relationships to each other. Confusion is disorientation, the term confusion being used especially when the patient is not aware that he is disoriented. This lack of awareness of confusion, this anosognosia, is the basis for calling a confusional state a psychosis, since the psychotic person by definition has a perverse and distorted relation to reality. Disorientation is ultimately the basis for all psychotic behavior of organic origin.

Dementia is defined as a more or less sustained, but not necessarily irreversible, decline from a previously attained intellectual level. It is not the same as psychosis although it may lead to psychosis. The difference between the nonpsychotic and the psychotic dement is again a matter of the patient's awareness of the intellectual defect. Dementia is not to be identified with cerebral atrophy, although a certain number of dements may have cerebral atrophy.

Much of modern psychology is concerned with the problem of finding least common denominators of normal and abnormal behavior. No formulation has yet succeeded in satisfying the physiologist, the physician, or the psychologist himself. As a result, the step from phenomenology to physiology is troublesome in the behavioral disorders. The best one can do, given the present development of our knowledge, is to identify the basic category of disordered function. All behavioral phenomena ultimately can be related to one or more of the following functional groups:

    Nonorganic psychological
    Perception, including
       gnosia
       spatiotemporal integration
       spatiomotor integration
    Abstraction
    Memory
    Prospection
    Language
    Regulation of emotional display

"Prospection" is a term submitted in embarrassment. It refers to the ability to predict what will happen in the future on the basis of what is happening in the present or has happened in the past. It is part of what some would call "judgment."

It is not possible in all cases to make easy transition from the physiological to the anatomical. This reflects the inadequacy of our knowledge of the very complex anatomy and physiology of the human nervous system. Disorders of perception, probably the largest of the physiological categories, may mean an anatomical locus at the periphery, or in the alerting mechanisms of the brain stem, or in the primary receptive areas of the cortex, or in the association areas, especially the posterior parietal regions. The capacity for abstraction is very difficult to localize; it may fail because perception is deranged, it may require intact memory, it is often impaired in seemingly pure frontal lesions. Memory defect is more clearly correlated with bilateral temporal, and probably specifically, hippocampal lesions. There have been some reports of unilateral basitemporal lesions that disrupt memory. It is possible that this can occur in very acute unilateral lesions. Victor, Adams, and Collins (1971) have shown that lesions in the medial dorsal thalamus are responsible for the severe memory loss of Korsakoff's dementia. The anatomical lesions of language disorders remain in the "quadrilateral space of Marie." Some may be unhappy about including the category of language in the analysis of behavioral disorders, but the patient with a sensory aphasia is denied the chance for normal interpersonal relationships with his fellows, and the patient with the full picture of a jargon aphasia must be considered psychotic by any standard. The regulation of emotional display may be disrupted by lesions in the limbic system, but in the most common example, the forced laughter and crying of pseudobulbar palsy, the lesions are widespread in frontobulbar connections and basal ganglia.

While keeping in mind that the lobar divisions of the human brain are highly arbitrary, it is clinically useful in a restricted way to know the general localizing features for the major subdivisions of the cerebral hemispheres. These are enumerated in Tables 1, 2, and 3. A basioccipital lesion has been described which produces a severe agitation, not infrequently fatal of itself. The complex effects of seizure discharges in the various parts of brain, and especially in the temporal lobe, must be kept in mind in any consideration

TABLE 1

Manifestations of Frontal Lobe Disease

Defects in judgment
Defects in planning for the future
Defects in relating present to past events
Absurd jocularity
Gait disturbance
Grasping phenomena
Gaze perseveration
Repetitive movements

TABLE 2

Manifestations of Temporal Lobe Disease

Psychomotor seizures
Memory defect
Confabulation
Lack of initiative
Emotional blandness
Hallucinations and delusions
Language disturbances

TABLE 3

Manifestations of Parietal Lobe Disease

Visuospatial and spatiomotor defects
Avoiding reflexes
Inattention to environmental stimuli
Confusion of sidedness
Hallucinations and delusions
Defective synthesis of complex sensory data
Anosognosia
Language disorders

of behavioral disorders.

Anatomically a distinction must be made between lesions *on* brain and *in* brain. Compression of a cerebral hemisphere from outside is diagnosed when a patient's alertness is reduced and failing, with or without hemiparesis or confusion, and in the absence of "deep" signs and cranial nerve signs other than those involving the third nerve. The most common cause of this is subdural hematoma. Lesions in the brain stem may produce stupor, apathy, and inattention which may go on to hallucinations of many different sorts, including those called "peduncular hallucinoses."

The clinician will be disappointed if he seeks "pure" anatomical syndromes in the behavioral changes of the elderly. Most often there is a mixture of symptoms and signs, reflecting the experience of the pathologist in finding that in the elderly many different parts of the brain are involved, whatever the nature of the lesion.

In the occurrence of very focal symptoms and signs one always looks for a focal lesion, but even the slowly progressing degenerative dementias may be initiated or punctuated by specific language disturbances, seizures, or other phenomena of high localizing value. Patterns of early development vary in the degenerative dementias. Although the most common presentation is a simple memory loss probably explained on the basis of early hippocampal involvement, there are other presentations of spatiomotor and visuospatial disorganization caused by parietooccipital involvement, or of errors in judgment caused by frontal involvement. The extent to which one pushes special diagnostic procedures depends in large part on the possibility of finding a focal remediable process. It is regrettable that so many unnecessary diagnostic procedures are being done on elderly patients. These procedures could be reduced in number by careful analysis of the clinical data used to attain physiological and anatomical diagnosis.

The Remediable or Preventable Lesions

The pathological diagnosis uses the data of the physiological and anatomical diagnoses but requires much more. The accumulation of additional data requires the high exercise of clinical judgment. An effective approach to pathological diagnosis can be made by considering first the remediable or preventable causes of confusion or dementia in the elderly person. There is no tragedy in failing to diagnose a bifrontal glioblastoma multiforme or Pick's disease, but it is a tragedy to miss myxedema, subdural hematoma, or hyponatremia. Every patient should be looked at from this point of view. The categories are listed in Table 4. There are other rare remediable causes in the elderly, such as nonconvulsive status epilepticus manifesting itself as a confusional state. Transient ischemic attacks rarely present as a pure behavioral change. A useful rule states that an acute confusional state in an elderly person is a *medical* emergency. It is, in almost all cases, the result of a process originating outside nervous tissue and altering the environment of nervous tissue without producing permanent structural change.

TABLE 4
Confusion and/or Dementia—the Remediable or Preventable Causes

Intoxications
Infections
Metabolic disorders
Nutritional defects
Subdural hematoma
Benign intracranial tumors
Occult hydrocephalus
Sensory deprivation

Causes of the intoxications include all drugs a physician may prescribe for a patient, all drugs the patient may get on his own across the counter, all chemicals a disenchanted wife or husband may slip into the diet, and, above all, alcohol. The abuse of alcohol by aged persons is much underestimated by the aged themselves and by physicians who do not include the question in the system review. The reduced adaptability of advanced age is nowhere better illustrated than in the aged person's decreased tolerance to dosages that in youth or middle age would have produced only minimal effect.

The infections that disorganize the elderly are not only the pyogenic and viral leptomeningitides, general paresis, and fungal diseases of the brain, but also the extracranial infections, as in lung or urinary tract, whose systemic manifestation so often is acute confusion with or without fever or septicemia.

The metabolic disorders range all the way. They include dehydration, electrolyte disturbances, hypo- and hyperthyroidism, hypoglycemia, nonketotic hyperosmolar states, diabetic acidosis, pulmonary insufficiency with hypoxia and hypercarbia, hepatic insufficiency, uremia, Addison's disease, and Cushing's disease.

There is no good information about the frequency of confusion and dementia due to malnutrition because so often the causes that predispose to malnutrition result from or predispose to other kinds of behavioral disorder. These causes range from depression to toothlessness, and they include some cases of absorption defect and alcoholism. Ever so often we still see a case of frank pellagra in the elderly person for whom food has lost its appeal.

Of the neurosurgically remediable lesions, subdural hematoma and benign tumor generally have some associated motor, sensory, and reflex disturbances. In the elderly, subdural hematoma may present only with a behavioral change, and it should be thought of especially in patients who have been on anticoagulants and have become lethargic or stuporous. The troublesome benign tumors are the olfactory groove meningiomas, the anterior parasagittal meningiomas, and the acoustic neuromas. Within the last year we have seen two patients in their late sixties who had behavioral changes relating to the endocrinopathy of their pituitary tumors. Occult hydrocephalus is a rare entity in its primary form, but sometimes occult hydrocephalus bespeaks an occult third-ventricle tumor or an acoustic neuroma.

Disease of the sensory organs or disease of the motor apparatus may produce a degree of sensory deprivation sufficient to produce disorientation and confusion in an elderly person.

The Irremediable Processes

The irremediable dementias can be thought of as vascular and nonvascular in origin. Too much emphasis has been placed on vascular disease as a cause of dementia, and the term arteriosclerotic dementia has been thrown about irresponsibly for too long. Actually there are very few circumstances in which dementia may result from vascular disease of the brain without overwhelming disease in motor, sensory, and reflex systems. Table 5 outlines the role of vascular disease in the production of dementia. Under the heading of strategically placed focal lesions one would include disturbances of language that can seriously affect behavior, like sensory aphasia and jargon aphasia.

It is convenient to think of the irremediable nonvascular dementias as being associated or not associated with movement disorders early in the course of the diseases. Table 6 outlines this approach. No attempt is made here to affirm or deny that Alzheimer's senile dementia is the same process as Alzheimer's presenile dementia. Those who feel strongly that these are different states argue that in the presenium the disease progresses more rapidly, has more focal symptoms and signs, and is associated more often with convulsive disorder. I am not sure these arguments are valid. The experienced clinician sees patients in the presenium who move slowly without seizures and focal change, and if he attends with the same intensity of concern and observation to patients in the senium, he will find instances of rapid progression, focal signs and seizures.

TABLE 5
The Role of Vascular Disease in Dementia

Multiple embolic or nonembolic infarcts
Strategically located infarcts
Diffuse ischemic encephalopathy
Disease of small arteries
    diabetes
    hypertension

TABLE 6
The Irremediable Nonvascular Dementias

With Movement Disorder	Without Movement Disorder
Huntington's chorea	Pick's
Creutzfeldt-Jakob disease	Alzheimer's
Wilson's disease	Senile brain atrophy
Progressive subcortical gliosis (Neumann and Cohn 1967)	Alzheimer's nonspecific (Schaumberg and Suzuki 1968)
Progressive supranuclear palsy	

Efforts have been made to distinguish clinically between Alzheimer's disease and Pick's disease but none of these efforts has been completely successful (Sjögren, Sjögren, and Lindgren 1952). The point has been made by many clinicians that the patient with Alzheimer's disease preserves at least the superficial appearances of social appropriateness. This is generally true, but it may be true of other dementing illnesses as well and exceptions are common within the Alzheimer group.

One caution must be noted in this otherwise useful distinction of the irremediable dementias on the basis of their association with movement disorders. There are a few cases of Alzheimer's disease in which myoclonus appears early in the disease (Jacob 1970). Late in the course, all patients with extensive cerebral involvement, including Alzheimer's disease, may develop myoclonus.

Compensation and Decompensation in the Nervous System

The concept of compensation and decompensation in other organs and tissues is familiar to all physicians, who speak easily and often about cardiac, pulmonary, renal, or hepatic decompensation. Although the principle is not evoked as often in disease of the brain, it is nevertheless an equally valid concept in nervous tissue. Compensation in an anatomically deranged organ or organ system indicates that function has been maintained or re-established despite the anatomical defect. The marvelous adaptability of the human nervous system allows compensation for many anatomical defects if they are not excessive in size or in number. Compensation is less easily attained as people grow older but it is never completely absent. The best illustrations of neurological compensation and decompensation may be seen in simple systems like optic nerve, but the principle still applies in the complex problems of behavior in the elderly. Table 7 lists some causes of decompensation of the elderly brain, as seen in the author's recent experience.

Even in patients with structurally irreversible lesions, there remains the possibility of improvement in a behavioral pattern by maintaining the patient's external and internal environment to allow as much compensation as possible for the underlying anatomical disorder. The objective may be a limited one, but for many patients this is the critical difference that may permit them to be at home rather than in an institution, to maintain some dignity even though a degree of dementia remains. The patient with senile dementia may decompensate only at night, or only when his bladder distends to produce painful discomfort, or only when he is fatigued or febrile. The good physician who follows the patient over a period of time begins to see patterns of environmental disorder, both internal and external, that lead to decompensation, and he changes those things that are in his power to change. The patient or his family frequently sees these episodes of decompensation as evidence of progressing disease; the physician must educate them, if they are educable, about the reasons for the fluctuations.

TABLE 7

Some Causes of Decompensation

Fatigue	Cardiac failure
Fever	Pulmonary insufficiency
Infection	Bladder distention
Dehydration	Intoxication
Electrolyte imbalance	Withdrawal
Trauma	Malnutrition
Seizures	Isolation

Treatment. Treatment then depends on analysis of the phenomenological, physiological, anatomical, and pathological diagnoses. Sometimes the symptom alone is treatable, as when a patient with nocturnal agitation requires a soporific drug. Sometimes the physiology can be altered, as in providing a hearing device to the deaf, paranoid, old man. The anatomy and physiology can be altered by removing a subdural hematoma over a hemisphere. The pathological process may be reversed by treating the underlying nutritional defect. The decompensating challenges can be identified and controlled. In some patients it is necessary to work one's therapy on the basis of all the diagnostic hierarchies.

References

Jacob, H. 1970. *Muscular Twitchings in Alzheimer's Disease, Alzheimer's Disease and Related Conditions.* G.E.W. Wolstenholme and M. O'Connor (eds.). London: Churchill.

Neumann, M.A., and Cohn, R. 1967. Progressive subcortical gliosis, a rare form of presenile dementia. *Brain* 90:405.

Schaumberg, H.H., and Suzuki, K. 1968. Non-specific familial presenile dementia. *J. Neurol. Neurosurg. Psychiat.* 31:479.

Sjögren, T.; Sjögren, H.; and Lindgren, A.G.H. 1952. Morbus Alzheimer and morbus Pick. *Acta Psychiat. Neurol. Scand.* suppl. 82.

Victor, M.; Adams, R.D.; and Collins, G.H. 1971. *Wernicke-Korsakoff Syndrome.* Philadelphia: Davis.

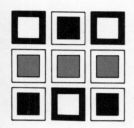

The Relationship Between Organic Brain Disease and Physical Status

Raymond Harris, M.D.

Subdepartment of Cardiovascular Medicine
St. Peter's Hospital, Albany, New York

> *"The mind is so intimately dependent upon the condition and relation of the organs of the body that if any means can ever be found to render man wiser and more ingenious than hitherto, I believe that it is in Medicine they must be sought for."*
>
> René Descartes

Is There a Relationship Between Organic Brain Disease and General Physical Status?

Numerous studies in the medical literature support a direct relationship in the elderly between poor physical status and organic brain disease with psychiatric impairment. Simon (1968) reported that four-fifths of 534 geriatric patients hospitalized primarily for chronic brain syndrome and senile brain disease also suffered physical impairments severe enough to interfere with their daily functions. In his series the most common physical illnesses, in descending order of frequency, were malnutrition, congestive heart failure, stroke, hypertension, serious respiratory infection, peripheral neuritis often associated with alcoholism, and cancer. Kay and Roth (1955) found 82 percent of the severely ill medical patients they studied in old age homes had moderate or severe brain syndromes. Hader, Schulman, and Faigman (1965) uncovered physical illness in 90 percent of the mentally ill patients they examined in a geriatric mental hygiene clinic.

The following nosological classification of chronic brain disorders, adapted from the American Psychiatric Association classification, quickly reviews the medical conditions associated with organic brain disorders (Table 1) and supports their intimate relationship.

163

TABLE 1

Chronic Brain Disorders Associated with:

1. Congenital cranial anomaly, congenital spastic paraplegia, Mongolism, prenatal maternal infectious disease, birth trauma
2. Central nervous system syphilis (meningoencephalitic)
3. Central nervous system syphilis (meningovascular)
4. Other central nervous system syphilis
5. Intracranial infection other than syphilis
6. Intoxication (lead, arsenic, mercury, carbon monoxide, illuminating gas, miscellaneous drugs, and alcohol)
7. Brain trauma
8. Cerebral arteriosclerosis
9. Circulatory disturbance other than cerebral arteriosclerosis (cerebral embolism, cerebral hemorrhage, arterial hypertension, and other chronic cardiovascular disease)
10. Convulsive disorder
11. Senile brain disease
12. Other disturbances of metabolism, growth, or nutrition (Alzheimer's disease, endocrine disorders, pellagra, familial amaurosis, avitaminosis)
13. Intracranial neoplasm
14. Diseases of unknown or uncertain cause (multiple sclerosis, Huntington's chorea, Pick's disease, and other diseases of a familial or hereditary nature)
15. Unknown cause

It is important for both the clinician and the psychiatrist to be fully aware of the increased incidence and severity of physical illness and disease in patients with psychiatric disorders, especially among the elderly whose bizarre psychiatric and behavioral alterations may be due to organic physical illness of the brain or other organs. Very often a heightened brain syndrome or psychiatric complaint in geriatric patients heralds severe physical illness (Hader, Schulman, and Faigman 1965). Mental symptoms of psychotic depression or organic brain disease may precede the clinical diagnosis of cancer (McGovern, Miller, and Robertson 1959) in patients with primary brain tumors, metastatic lesions to the brain, or even in the absence of demonstrable cerebral metastases, meningeal infiltration, peripheral neuropathy, or myopathy (Posner 1971). Psychiatric disturbances associated with carcinoma in the absence of demonstrable metastatic deposits in the brain occur most often in patients with lung carcinoma, ovarian and breast cancer, and less often with other tumors.

In addition to cancer, other illnesses, particularly cardiovascular and pulmonary conditions, may aggravate or predispose toward the development of chronic organic brain disease (Table 2). As a cardiologist I see many patients who consult me primarily for heart disease but who also show disturbing signs and symptoms of early organic brain disease which render management of their heart condition more difficult (Harris 1970 and 1971).

In my practice, patients with pulmonary disease also display mental symptoms simulating organic brain disease. One such patient was T.H., an elderly man whose psychiatrist gave him electric shock therapy when his brain symptoms were actually due to hypoxia (Table 3).

Possible Mechanisms Relating Organic Brain Disease and Physical Status

The title of my paper gives me license to discuss the possible mechanisms by which poor physical status causes, predisposes toward, or aggravates organic brain disease in aging patients.

As Delgado (1969) points out, "A common error in science is to try to simplify the observed phenomenon and to reduce causality to a single factor, excluding all other variables. This is the fallacy of the single cause or failure to understand that a biological phenomenon is always the product of a complex situation, not of a single determinant." Likewise, there is no *simple*, single relationship between physical status and organic brain disease. Utilizing a schema proposed by Delgado (1969), however, the presumptive relationship between physical status and organic brain disease may be analyzed in terms of three major dynamic components: *Sensory input*, which is determined by environmental circumstances perceived through sensory receptors and acting upon the individual; *throughput*, which is the personal processing of these environmental circumstances through the intracerebral mechanisms established by genetic endowment and enhanced by previous experiences; and *output*, represented by individual and social behavior which, for the subject of this paper, constitutes the observable manifestations of chronic organic brain disease.

Sensory Input

Many investigators believe that behavior, to a considerable degree, consists of an automatic response to sensory inputs and that change in sensory input affects a patient's behavior. Aging patients may sustain an involuntary reduction in sensory input as the result of the aging process or disease which interferes with their ability to hear, see, taste, smell, adapt to light, and perceive color. Such sensory impairments, when severe, may initiate reverberations in the psychological sphere and induce personality changes (Busse 1965).

Experimental reduction of sensory input has provoked psychological disturbances like hallucinations, distortions of the body image, and severe anxiety in aging patients with chronic organic brain disease and even in some healthy individuals. Cameron (1941), for example, demonstrated in senile patients with nocturnal deliria that delirious states can be reproduced in the daytime by placing the patient in a dark room. Ziskind et al. (1960) showed that the application of eye patches to both eyes of patients after cataracts had been removed produced delirioid symptoms in elderly patients with demonstrable or subclinical organic impairment of brain function. The elderly patient's lack of ability to

TABLE 2

Causes of Metabolic Brain Disease

I. Deprivation of Oxygen, Substrate, or Metabolic Cofactors
   *A. Hypoxia (interference with oxygen supply to the entire brain — cerebral blood flow normal)
      1. Decreased oxygen tension and content of blood
            Pulmonary disease
            Alveolar hypoventilation
            Decreased atmospheric oxygen tension
      2. Decreased oxygen content of blood — normal tension
            Anemia
            Carbon monoxide poisoning
            Methemoglobinemia
   *B. Ischemia (diffuse or widespread multifocal interference with blood supply to brain)
      1. Decreased cerebral blood flow resulting from decreased cardiac output
            Stokes-Adams syndrome, cardiac arrest, cardiac arrhythmias
            Myocardial infarction
            Congestive heart failure
            Aortic stenosis
      2. Decreased cerebral blood flow resulting from decreased peripheral resistance in systemic
         circulation
            Syncope: orthostatic, vasovagal
            Carotid sinus hypersensitivity
            Low blood volume
      3. Decreased cerebral blood flow due to generalized increase in cerebrovascular resistance
            Hypertensive encephalopathy
            Hyperventilation syndrome
            Increased blood viscosity (polycythemia), cryo- and macroglobinemia
      4. Decreased local cerebral blood flow due to widespread small vessel occlusion
            Disseminated intravascular coagulation
            Systemic lupus erythematosus
            Subacute bacterial endocarditis
   *C. Hypoglycemia
            Resulting from exogenous insulin
            Spontaneous (endogenous insulin, liver disease, etc.)
    D. Cofactor deficiency
            Thiamin (Wernicke's encephalopathy)
            Niacin
            Pyridoxine
            B_{12}

II. Diseases of Organs Other than Brain
   *A. Diseases of nonendocrine organs
            Liver (hepatic coma)
            Kidney (uremic coma)
            Lung (CO_2 narcosis)
   *B. Hyper- and/or hypofunction of endocrine organs
            Pituitary
            Thyroid (myxedema-thyrotoxicosis)
            Parathyroid (hyper- and hypoparathyroidism)
            Adrenal (Addison's disease, Cushing's disease, pheochromocytoma)
            Pancreas (diabetes, hypoglycemia)

TABLE 2

Causes of Metabolic Brain Disease *(continued)*

C. Water and electrolyte imbalance
      Hypo-osmolality (water intoxication)
      Hyperosmolality (nonketotic diabetic coma)
      Hyper- and hypocalcemia

III. Exogenous Poisons
  *A. Sedative drugs
  B. Acid poisons or poisons with acidic breakdown products
      Paraldehyde
      Methyl alcohol
      Ethylene glycol
  C. Other enzyme inhibitors
      Heavy metals
      Organic phosphates
      Cyanide
      Salicylates
  D. Others
      Penicillin
      Anticonvulsants
      Steroids
      Cardiac glycosides

IV. Diseases Producing Toxins or Enzyme Inhibition in CNS
  A. Meningitis
  B. Encephalitis
  C. Subarachnoid hemorrhage

V. Abnormalities of Ionic or Acid-Base Environment of CNS
  A. Water and sodium (hyper- and hyponatremia)
  B. Acidosis (metabolic and respiratory)
  C. Alkalosis (metabolic and respiratory)
  D. Potassium (hyper- and hypokalemia)
  E. Magnesium (hyper- and hypomagnesemia)
  F. Calcium (hyper- and hypocalcemia)

VI. Miscellaneous Diseases of Unknown Cause
  A. Sepsis
  B. Febrile states
  C. Seizures and postictal states
  D. "Postoperative" delirium
  E. Concussion

* Alone or in combination, the most common causes of delirium seen on general medical wards.

From Cecil-Loeb *Textbook of Medicine*, 13th Edition, 1971. Reprinted with permission of the author, Jerome B. Posner; publisher, W.B. Saunders Company, Philadelphia; editor, Walsh McDermott.

TABLE 3

Arterial Blood Gases

Date	Time	pH	pCO$_2$(mm Hg)	pO$_2$(mm Hg)	% O$_2$ Sat.
7/3	(admission)	7.34	76	.36	67
7/3	11:30 p.m.	7.31	69	78	96
7/4	9 a.m.	7.25	79	40	
	1 p.m.	7.24	72.5	55	87
	7 p.m.	7.22	82	64	
	9:30 p.m.	Endotracheal tube inserted			
7/5	2 a.m.	7.48	50		97
7/7		7.4	47.5	54	87
		Tracheostomy			

Table 3 shows arterial blood gas changes in 65-year-old man (T.H.) hospitalized with chronic pulmonary emphysema, chronic cor pulmonale, heart failure, and acute ventilatory failure. Prior to admission, his psychiatrist gave him electroshock because of mental symptoms suggesting psychiatric illness. He was very drowsy and lethargic on admission. Treatment on admission included tracheal and bronchial suction, administration of oxygen by Venturi mask, saturated solution of potassium iodide (SSKI), tetracycline, digitalis, and diuretics. Between 1 and 7 p.m. on 7/4, 1,000 cc of 5-percent glucose in water, 500 mg of aminophylline, and nasal oxygen were given. Because of progressive clinical deterioration of the patient and of his arterial blood gases and pH, an endotracheal tube was inserted at 9:30 p.m. Assisted mechanical ventilation with Bird respirator was begun. Tracheostomy became necessary on 7/7. Patient improved and was eventually discharged from the hospital. He remained free from mental symptoms and returned to his regular work.

From Harris, R. 1970. *The Management of Geriatric Cardiovascular Disease.* Reprinted with permission of the publisher, J.B. Lippincott, Philadelphia.

adapt to the dark and his decreased perception of various levels of illumination explain why elderly people may become anxious and disturbed when moving from a well-lit to a dark room.

Voluntary decrease of sensory imput by a deliberate unwillingness on the part of the older person to make an effort or to socialize presents a more complicated situation. The barrage of sensory stimuli with which elderly people are acoustically assaulted by radio and optically by television, literature, news media, propaganda, and advertisements may be one cause of a voluntary decrease in sensory input. In self-defense, older people may voluntarily "turn off" their sensory input, inhibit the processing of sensory stimuli, and refuse to use their minds despite the well-recognized fact that the normal development and function of the mind depends upon continuing healthy sensory input, productive thinking, and curiosity. As Samuel Johnson once noted, "Curiosity is one of the permanent and certain characteristics of a vigorous mind." Social, economic, and other problems stemming from the stereotyped responses of society to aging people may cause them voluntarily to withdraw and disengage from society, thereby further decreasing their sensory input and accelerating their mental deterioration.

Throughput

Throughput — the personal processing of those circumstances through which the intracerebral mechanism is laid down by genetic endowments and enhanced by experience — is most affected by alterations in brain function attributable to (1) neuronal changes, (2) reduced cerebral blood supply, (3) cerebral oxygenation, and (4) metabolic disorders affecting the brain.

Neuronal changes. There are characteristic gross and microscopic alterations in the normal aging brain. The weight of the brain is maximum by about age 20 to 25, and then regresses linearly seven to eleven percent between the ages of 20 to 96. Narrowed convolutions and widened sulci characteristic of the senile brain are structural changes associated with this weight loss.

Microscopically there are loss of neurons and increase in glial elements. The neuronal loss, uneven in distribution, is most marked in the temporal gyrus, less marked in the precentral gyrus and visual cortex, and least marked in the postcentral gyrus (Brody 1970). The cerebral cortex of the normal young adult human being is estimated to contain about 10 to 12 billion neurons. After the brain reaches its maximum brain weight at 20 years of age, it is estimated that 100,000 neurons are lost each day and the brain decreases in size and weight (Brody 1971). If this irreversible loss of nervous tissue with aging continues long enough, intellectual defects may be expected to develop. However, since intellectual defects are not always evident in many elderly persons, it appears that the brain may be able to compensate for the gradual loss of neurons (Busse 1965).

In addition to the loss of neurons with age, the pathologic causes of brain damage already listed in Tables 1 and 2 may also interfere with the function of the throughput and intracerebral mechanisms. I wish to focus attention on the more important causes such as cerebral blood supply, cerebral oxygenation, and metabolic disorders.

Cerebral blood supply. A reasonably normal cerebral blood flow appears essential to maintain the integrity of the intracerebral mechanism or the throughput. The ordinary changes in the cerebral blood flow with aging are insufficient to cause significant brain disease, but a reduced cerebral blood flow as a result of cardiovascular disease may interfere with the cellular function of the brain cells and cause organic brain disease. Kety (1960) demonstrated a significant decrease in cerebral blood flow and oxygen consumption of the brain in patients with cerebral arteriosclerosis and senile psychosis as compared with values in healthy young men. The decreased cerebral blood flow in these patients is the result of increased cerebrovascular resistance which is about twice the normal value and represents a physiological confirmation during life of the well-known sclerotic changes observed in these brains postmortem.

Butler's study of cerebral circulation and metabolism revealed no significant difference in cerebral blood flow and oxygen consumption between normal young subjects (mean age 21 years) and elderly healthy men (mean age 71 years). Any reduction in cerebral blood flow occurred in subjects with evidence of arteriosclerosis, suggesting that decreased cerebral blood flow and oxygen consumption in older people are not the consequence of chronologic aging per se, but rather of arteriosclerosis which causes first relative cerebral circulatory insufficiency and hypoxia, and ultimately a secondary reduction in cerebral metabolic rate. Cerebral arteriosclerosis with consequent reduction in cerebral blood flow and oxygen consumption may be one pathway leading to senility. Some patients with early senile manifestations in Butler's study, however, had neither clinically diagnosable arteriosclerosis nor evidence of cerebral circulatory or metabolic changes. Although both senility and arteriosclerosis occur fairly commonly in old age, these conditions may not bear any essential pathogenic relationship to each other (Butler 1963).

A more recent study by Ingvar and Gustafson (1971), using the xenon[133] clearance technique, attributed reduced regional cerebral blood flow in 38 patients with organic dementia of early onset to a metabolic disorder with decreased metabolic demand and secondary blood flow reduction caused primarily by degenerative cellular changes.

Acute mental confusion in elderly people with congestive heart failure may result from reduced cerebral blood flow proportionate to the fall in cardiac output and the increase in cerebral vasoconstriction. Cardiac arrhythmias may also decrease cerebral blood flow and produce cerebral ischemia. The most dramatic example is cardiac arrest which cuts off the blood supply to the brain and causes permanent brain damage or death if cardiac resuscitation is delayed too long.

Frequent premature ventricular contractions in animals, and presumably in patients, may reduce the cerebral blood flow 12 to 25 percent. Frequent premature atrial systoles may reduce cerebral blood flow approximately 8 percent. Atrial tachycardia or atrial flutter fibrillation with a rapid ventricular rate may lower cerebral blood flow by 20 to 40 percent. Reduced cerebral blood flow also has been demonstrated in patients with complete atrioventricular block. Correction of the bradycardia by electrical pacing improves cerebral blood flow and prevents further brain damage in some patients. In patients with cerebral vascular disease and supraventricular tachycardia, cardioversion of cardiac arrhythmias to normal sinus rhythm almost always increases cardiac output and cerebral blood flow (Cooper and West 1970).

Stroke, a common cause of organic brain disease, is due usually to cerebral hemorrhage, thrombosis, or emboli, but some strokes in patients with atrial fibrillation may be produced by poor cerebral perfusion pressure rather than embolism, as a result of a fall in cardiac output and cerebral blood flow. Some strokes in patients after an acute myocardial infarction may be due to the dislodging of mural thrombi with resulting cerebral emboli, or as recent studies show, to a combination of cerebral atherosclerosis and poor cerebral perfusion (Cooper and West 1970).

Extracranial arterial disease is not a frequent cause of chronic psychosis in patients with organic brain syndrome. In an unselected psychiatric hospital population, 23 of 100 psychotic patients over the age of 45 with arteriographic visualization showed evidence of extracranial cerebral vascular disease. Only 7 showed advanced or total obstruction of the carotid or vertebral arteries, and there was no improvement in 4 patients in whom reconstructive arterial surgery was performed successfully (Bryant et al. 1965).

Trauma can also precipitate a stroke by causing traumatic thrombosis of the carotid artery. A blow to the neck may initiate a thrombotic process in the cervical portion of an atherosclerotic carotid artery and produce a stroke six weeks later. Sudden angulation of the head may also traumatize the internal carotid artery where it passes over bony prominences and cause a stroke (Clinical Pathological Conference 1971).

Older individuals with mild to moderate hypertension seem less vulnerable to organic brain disease, probably because the increased blood pressure increases cerebral blood flow, thereby compensating for impaired cerebral vascular autoregulation. Diastolic blood pressures above 106 mm Hg, however, may be associated with intellectual decline (Busse 1971). Drugs lowering high blood pressure may sometimes aggravate mental symptoms in elderly people in whom absentmindedness and other early signs of organic cerebral disease are already clinically apparent.

Cerebral oxygenation. Arterial blood oxygen tension decreases with age, even in the absence of known cardiopulmonary disease. The normal arterial blood oxygen tension in healthy persons over the age of 60 may fall to 65 to 80 mm Hg as compared with the normal values of 95 to 105 mm Hg partial oxygen pressure (pO_2) under the age of 30 (Harris 1970). There is little evidence, however, that the psychological symptoms of senescence arise from this relative hypoxia of brain tissue, although a body of experimental evidence reveals that hypoxia produces functional changes in the brain which in some respects resemble those occurring spontaneously in advanced aging (Gordon 1971). Most controlled studies relating oxygen supply to cognitive function have involved the effects of *acutely* induced hypoxia on the learned behavior of trained laboratory animals. These studies indicate that recent memory and learning are particularly sensitive to acute oxygen deprivation.

As far as chronic oxygen deprivation is concerned, the work of Jacobs et al. (1969) in 13 elderly male patients with *chronic* cognitive defects, treated with 30 intermittent exposures to 100 percent oxygen at 2.5 atmospheres in a hyperbaric chamber, are most provocative and encouraging. A large increase in arterial blood oxygen tension was found among the experimental subjects, while negligible changes were found among control patients. Psychological tests of cognitive function after treatment showed highly significant gains over pretreatment levels in the treated patients, suggesting the improved performance after therapy persisted beyond a temporary increase in arterial blood oxygen tension levels. This study suggests that high oxygen input affects the oxygen delivery system at some point and influences the function of tissue assumed to be marginally hypoxic (Jacobs et al. 1969). Although similar experiments at the Mount Sinai Hospital failed to confirm these results, further investigation of hyperbaric oxygen therapy is warranted in patients with chronic organic brain disease.

Further evidence of the importance of hypoxia as a cause of brain disease is suggested by the results of psychological tests of 100 patients with chronic obstructive pulmonary disease at the University of Nebraska. This study disclosed a high percentage of patients with early organic brain dysfunction related primarily to minor hemisphere functions such as visual coordination, eye-motor coordination, and visual integration (Innes et al. 1971). Of the three instruments used to assess the brain damage, namely the Wechsler Adult Intelligence Scale, Hooper, and Benton tests, 88.2 percent of the patients showed evidence of brain dysfunction on at least one of these tests, 52.7 percent on two of the three tests, and 12.9 percent on all three tests.

Chronic carbon monoxide poisoning may also interfere with the throughput intracerebral mechanism. Such ecological poisoning is frequently encountered because of the steadily increasing use of gasoline engines and the spread of air pollution (Gilbert and Glaser 1959). Patients with this disorder may show symptoms of anoxia or organic brain syndrome of fluctuating severity. The most common symptoms or complaints include anorexia, nausea, weight loss, apathy, fatigability, headache, dizziness, insomnia, and personality disturbances. Other symptoms may be palpitations, impaired memory, diminished tolerance to alcohol, ataxia, and unconsciousness. Policemen and workers in closed automobile garages are prime suspects for chronic organic brain disease produced by chronic carbon monoxide poisoning. Even farmers are not exempt. Of 30 cases of chronic carbon monoxide asphyxia collected by Katz (1958), 6 occurred in farmers operating tractors.

Metabolic disorders affecting the brain. Organic brain disease associated with diabetes, disorders of the thyroid, pituitary, and adrenal glands, and other medical conditions have been noted in Tables 1 and 2.

Elderly diabetics often develop symptoms and signs of organic brain disease as a result of cerebral arteriosclerosis or hypoglycemia. Although overdose of insulin is the most common cause of hypoglycemia, even one tablet of an oral antidiabetic agent, such as Diabinese, may produce hypoglycemia and permanent brain damage in elderly patients with poor food intake. Dehydration and its resultant hyperosmolarity in patients with advanced diabetes may produce dysfunction of cerebral hemispheres and the brain stem activating mechanisms, leading to further signs and symptoms of organic brain disease. Middle-aged and elderly diabetics should always be tested to determine their capacity for registration, memory, and constructional ability to make sure they know how to follow their doctor's instructions and to take their medications.

A study by Reitan (1967) demonstrates that a 10-percent or greater reduction of serum cholesterol in older men, even when the initial level is not markedly elevated, preserves psychologic functions which otherwise deteriorate with known cerebral damage or age. Reitan gave orally one-half ounce of 20-percent suspension of sitosterols three times daily before meals to elderly patients whose serum cholesterol levels averaged 240 mg per 100 mm or more during a preceding control period. The patients whose cholesterol levels were lowered showed the greatest absolute psychologic improvement of any of the four groups retested after twelve months of therapy. Confirmation of these results seems important since it is one of the few studies demonstrating how better control of natural elements in the blood will retard psychologic changes presumably related to brain changes with aging.

Deficiencies in thiamine, vitamin-B complex, and/or vitamin C may affect brain metabolism. The utilization of glucose by nerve cells requires the enzymatic action of certain vitamins, particularly vitamin B_1. When these vitamins are deficient, oxygenation cannot occur, creating conditions analogous to those in patients with hypoxia and associated with confusional states which usually disappear or improve with appropriate vitamin therapy. Such vitamin deficiencies may develop in old people subsisting on too much tea, bread, and water, and too little vegetables and fresh meat. Deficiencies of vitamin-B complex, vitamin B_{12}, and other vitamins may follow increased excretion after profound diuresis or elevated metabolism during infections.

Folic-acid or vitamin-B_{12} deficiencies may also be associated with a confusional state often mistakenly attributed to organic brain disease. Vitamin-B_{12} deficiencies may induce mental impairment in patients with pernicious anemia (Mitra 1971), alcoholism, or after the administration of tetracycline or isoniazid. Disorders due to folic-acid or vitamin-B_{12} deficiency do not always respond to therapy with these vitamins.

Amyloidosis involving the heart, aorta, and pancreatic islets may be found in patients with Alzheimer's disease (Schwartz 1971). Cerebral and cardiovascular amyloid deposits and amyloid degeneration of Langerhans' islets constitute a characteristic pathoanatomic triad in patients with senile mental and physical deterioration. Although immunobiologic mechanisms appear responsible for the formation of these amyloid deposits, tuberculosis should always be considered in the differential diagnosis of amyloidosis. A congophilic (amyloid?) material may be deposited in the brain and cause severe and permanent mental changes within hours or days after a catastrophic illness like subarachnoid hemorrhage, head injury, or cardiac surgery (Hollander and Strich 1970).

Output

"Time past and time future
What might have been and what has been
Point to one end, which is always present."
                                    T.S. Eliot, Four Quartets

The output or behavior of any person, as T.S. Eliot infers, is the product of a wide-ranging spectrum of past experiences, current sensory input, and functional biochemical processes in the brain. The output permits the physician and psychiatrist to diagnose organic brain disease in patients with classic disturbances of normal mental function. The diagnosis of organic brain disease presents little difficulty when the mental symptoms are accompanied by typical neurologic signs or the illness begins with fits, hemiplegia, or aphasia. When mental symptoms unfold gradually, however, exhibiting a vaguely neurotic or depressive quality without definite signs on physical examination, the condition has to be distinguished from psychoneurosis or an affective disorder (Barron and McMillan 1965).

A thorough physical examination is indicated in every patient with psychiatric problems before mental symptoms are attributed to purely psychiatric causes. Acute mental symptoms may be the first indication of unrecognized medical disease. Systematic examination of heart, lungs, and other organs should be performed to determine whether symptoms and signs are due to primary dysfunction of the brain or to dysfunction secondary to disease elsewhere. In patients whose symptoms are of relatively short duration, a minor head injury and/or chronic subdural hematoma should be considered. Patients should be queried about heart disease, gastrointestinal bleeding or hemorrhages, surgical operations, the type of anesthesia used, and the duration of anesthesia and recovery therefrom, the extent of any complications, and duration of bed rest after operation. A dietary and alcoholic beverage history should be taken. The diabetic patient should be asked about the frequency of hypoglycemic reactions, the dose of insulin, and the administration of oral antihyperglycemic agents. Obscure mental symptoms may be due to drugs in heart patients (Harris 1971) or to occult cancer, or hepatic insufficiency even in the absence of jaundice, splenomegaly, ascites, or other gross signs. Occult neoplasm and other medical conditions should not be ruled out in middle-aged and elderly subjects admitted for observation in mental hospitals and suffering from organic reactions (Charatan and Brierley 1956). Patients with iron deficiency or other types of anemia may also present with mental symptoms.

In addition to the usual medical and psychiatric evaluation, the diagnosis, evaluation, and treatment of elderly patients should pay attention to disturbances of sensory input, throughput, and output, and to the patient's physical condition, sensory deficits, social deprivation, and socioeconomic status. Specific dimensions of organization of daily activity, maintenance of goals in living and maintenance of social contacts, as well as a summary score of social responsiveness, may be associated significantly with one or more physiologic measures of cerebral blood flow, cerebral oxygen consumption, and cerebral glucose consumption (Butler 1963).

Improving Organic Brain Disease by Improving the Physical Status

Rational therapy to retard organic brain disease should include measures to improve the sensory inputs and physical status of older people. The patient's environment should be optimal for learning (Inskip 1970), offering sufficient visual, auditory, and tactile stimuli, so that even the patient with limited input becomes more sensitive to his external environment. Older people should have easy and unlimited access to centers of learning and thinking to improve their sensory input, and avoid limitations and regimentation that reduce learning experiences. Psychotherapy should improve the insight of aging people into their problems arising from aging and their relationship with the world.

In addition, any medical condition should be appropriately treated. Physical activity and exercise to improve muscle strength, endurance, mobility, and cardiovascular fitness, and to increase sensory input and recharge psychic and physical energies will help patients with organic brain disease. Ergotherapy (occupational therapy helping the aged to use the capacities they still possess) is one of the most basic treatments at the disposal of psychiatry and medicine to elevate the spirits of patients and diminish their sense of uselessness. Ludotherapy (treatment by games) helps the aged person who exhibits a tendency to disengage from the world and society. Kinesitherapy, associating the mobilization of the muscles with the psychological stimulation of recovered movements, tends to renew the body image and improve physical relations with the environment.

Sociotherapy should not be overlooked in the therapeutic management of patients with senile dementia (Villa and Ciompi 1968). Improvement of psychological functioning in patients with organic brain disease requires an environment in which the patient can function effectively within his intellectual and psychological capacity. The presence of familiar objects often facilitates orientation and reassures the elderly patient with a spotty memory. The sight of a familiar object — his pipe, hat, slippers, pillow, or the same bed, room, and house he has known in the past — often enables the patient who has been disoriented during a hospital stay to improve significantly at home (Tobis, Lowenthal, and Maringer 1957).

Some patients with mild chronic organic brain disease may have their years of independent functioning in the community prolonged by protective environmental manipulation, good general hygiene, and specific or symptomatic medical care. Such persons may maintain personal comfort by compulsive routine or well-automatized emotional habits and they readily respond to socially protective measures (Fisch et al. 1968).

Summary

In summary, the evidence indicates that a patient's organic brain disease is related to his general physical status. Measures to improve the general physical status may assist the aging patient with organic brain disease to attain better health and to live a more normal, happier, more productive, and independent life.

References

Barron, D.W., and McMillan, T.M. 1965. Office evaluation of the geriatric mental patient. *GP* 32:106.

Brody, H. 1970. Structural changes in the aging nervous system. In *Interdisciplinary Topics in Gerontology*, vol. 7. H.T. Blumenthal (ed.). New York: S. Karger, p. 9.

Brody, H. 1971. Personal communication.

Bryant, L.R.; Eiseman, B.; Spencer, F.C.; and Lieber, A. 1965. Frequency of extracranial cerebrovascular disease in patients with chronic psychosis. *New Eng. J. Med.* 272:12.

Busse, E.W. 1965. The early detection of aging. *Bull. N.Y. Acad. Med.* 41:1090.

Busse, E.W. 1971. Hyperbaric O_2 may keep elderly alert. *Internal Medicine News* 4:1, 28.

Butler, R.N. 1963. The facade of chronological age: an interpretative summary. *Amer. J. Psychiat.* 119:721.

Cameron, D.E. 1941. Studies in senile nocturnal delirium. *Psychiatric Quart.* 15:47.

Charatan, F.B., and Brierly, J.B. 1956. Mental disorder associated with primary lung carcinoma. *Brit. Med. J.* 1:765.

Clinical Pathological Conference 1971. Violence and the Brain. *JAMA* 216:1025.

Cooper, E.S., and West, J.W. 1970. Cardiac arrhythmias, cerebral function, and stroke. *Current Concepts of Cerebrobascular Disease and Stroke* 5:53.

Delgado, J.M.R. 1969. *Physical Control of the Mind — Toward a Psychocivilized Society.* New York: Harper & Row.

Descartes, R. *Discours de la Méthode*, Part VI. Trans. by J. Veitch. *Medical Tribune* (June 9) 1971, p. 9.

Eliot, T.S. 1943. *Four Quartets.* New York: Harcourt, Brace & World.

Fisch, M.; Goldfarb, A.I.; Shahinian, S.P.; and Turner, H. 1968. Chronic brain syndrome in the community aged. *Arch. Gen. Psychiat.* 18:739.

Gilbert, G.J., and Glaser, G.H. 1959. Neurologic manifestations of chronic carbon monoxide poisoning. *New Eng. J. Med.* 261:1217.

Gordon, P. 1971. *Advances in Gerontological Research*, vol. 3, p. 199. B.A. Strehler (ed.). New York: Academic Press.

Hader, M.; Schulman, P.M.; and Faigman, I. 1965. Heightened brain syndromes as precursors of severe physical illness in geriatric patients. *Amer. J. Psychiat.* 121:1124.

Harris, R. 1970. *The Management of Geriatric Cardiovascular Disease.* Philadelphia: J.B. Lippincott, p. 149.

Harris, R. 1971. Special features of heart disease in the elderly patient. In *Working with Older People*, vol. 4. A. Chinn (ed.). Washington, D.C.: U.S. Dept. of Health, Education and Welfare, Public Health Publication no. 1459.

Ingvar, D.H., and Gustafson, L. 1971. Regional cerebral blood flow in organic dementia with early onset. *Geriatrics Digest* 8:33 (Jan.).

Innes, R.J.; Sasser, M.A.; Strider, F.D.; and Wood, W.D. 1971. Psychological aspects of emphysema: Organic brain dysfunctions. Personal communication.

Inskip, W. 1970. Treatment programs for patients with chronic brain syndrome can be successful. *J. Amer. Geriat. Soc.* 18:631.

Jacobs, E.A.; Winter, P.M.; Alvis, H.J.; and Small, S.M. 1969. Hyperoxygenation effect on cognitive functioning in the aged. *New Eng. J. Med.* 281:753.

Katz, M. 1958. Carbon monoxide asphyxia: common clinical entity. *Canad. Med. Assoc. J.* 78:182.

Kay, D.W.K., and Roth, M. 1955. Physical illness and post-mortem findings in relation to different psychiatric groups aged 60 and over admitted to a county mental hospital. In *Old Age in the Modern World.* Edinburgh: E.S. Livingston.

Kety, S. 1960. The cerebral circulation. In *Handbook of Physiology,* vol. 3, chap. 71. Washington, D.C.: American Physiological Society, p. 1751.

McGovern, G.P.; Miller, D.H.; and Robertson, E.E. 1959. A mental syndrome associated with lung carcinoma. *Arch. Neurol. Psychiat.* 81:341.

Mitra, M.L. 1971. Confusional states in relation to vitamin deficiencies in the elderly. *J. Amer. Geriat. Soc.* 19:536.

Posner, J.B. 1971. Delirium and exogenous metabolic brain disease. In Cecil-Loeb *Textbook of Medicine.* P.B. Beeson and W. McDermott (eds.). 13th Ed. Philadelphia: W.B. Saunders, p. 88.

Posner, J.B. 1971. Nonmetastatic effects of cancer on the nervous system. In Cecil-Loeb *Textbook of Medicine.* P.B. Beeson and W. McDermott (eds.). 13th Ed. Philadelphia: W.B. Saunders, p. 288.

Reitan, R.M. 1967. Psychologic changes associated with aging and with cerebral damage. *Mayo Clinic Proceedings* 42:653.

Schwartz, P. 1971. Amyloidosis: Cause and manifestation of senile deterioration. *Geriatrics Digest* 8:20 (Feb.).

Simon, A. 1968. The geriatric mentally ill. *Gerontologist* 8 (II):7.

Tobis, J.S.; Lowenthal, M.; and Maringer, S. 1957. Evaluation and management of the brain-damaged patient. *JAMA* 165:2035.

Villa, J.L., and Ciompi, L. 1968. Therapeutic problems of senile dementia. In *Senile Dementia.* C. Muller and L. Ciompi (eds.). Bern: Hans Huber Publishers, p. 107.

Ziskind, E.; Jones, H.; Filante, W.; and Goldberg, J. 1960. Observations on mental symptoms in eye patched patients: hypnagogic symptoms in sensory deprivation. *Amer. J. Psychiat.* 116:893.

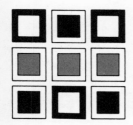

Multidimensional Treatment Approaches

Alvin I. Goldfarb, M.D.

Mount Sinai School of Medicine
of the City University of New York
New York, New York

Treatment of disorders is usually directed at causes or symptoms; it is specific or general. This requires discussion of what we mean by the aging brain and how it affects function.

The Aged Brain

In other chapters in this volume detailed attention is paid to the neurochemistry as well as the macro- and micropathology of the aged brain. The similarity between so-called senile brain changes and Alzheimer's disease has been stressed. Coincidentally, the problem of so-called cerebral arteriosclerosis—a condition that is not arteriosclerotic and need not necessarily involve large vessels in the cerebrum—has been touched upon. Agreed upon is the fact that the mark of aging in the brain is decreased brain weight and the loss of neurons, and that the neuronal loss is widespread throughout the cortex of the cerebral hemispheres as well as elsewhere in the brain.

The Aging Process

It is not clear whether senescent brain changes that lead to diffuse neuronal loss and decrease in brain weight with minimal neurofibrillary tangles and senile plaques differ qualitatively or simply quantitatively from the process called Alzheimer's disease. To clinicians it seems clear that the psychiatric syndrome characterized by disorientation for time, place, person, and situation, memory loss, decrease in information, and ability to calculate reflects brain cell loss or "damage." It appears also that such brain damage may be the result of a number of factors that act upon the brain, alone or in combination, some early and others late in the lifetime (Table 1).

179

TABLE 1

The Presumptive Relationship of Etiologic Factors to Acquired Intellectual Deficit and Associated "Functional" Disorders in the Aged

Multiple Etiology →	Brain Disturbance →	Manifestations →	Psychiatric Syndrome
Early and late physical factors: genetic accidents illness poisons	Cerebral malsupport (reversible=acute) Cerebral damage (irreversible=chronic)	Disorientation of time place person situation Memory loss recent remote Decrease in general information and intellectual functioning	Organic mental syndromes (acute brain syndrome— chronic brain syndrome) (measured by tests which reflect brain-cell loss [damage or dysfunction])
Situational experiential factors: family peers schooling occupation finances residence culture health and habits Personality factors: phenotype social ascriptions social achievements education occupation patterns of psychological emotional physical	Interpersonal friction Disorders of thinking behavior affect	Reaction to loss of intellect Search for aid and support elaborated as: apathy pseudoanhedonia display of helplessness somatization hypochondriasis depression paranoid states explotive-manipulative states	Modification of life-long well-established mechanisms of psychological, emotional, social, and physical adjustment Behavior disorder or "neurosis" or, if genetic, diathesis and phenotypical propensity "Psychotic" disorder with signs of parasympathomimetic or sympathomimetic vegetative signs

Table 1 attempts to show some of the etiologic or sequential relationships in the emergence of brain syndrome. It illustrates, moving from left to right, how factors or processes beginning early or late in a lifetime go on to influence the support of central nervous tissue with, at first, manifestations of poor cerebral function and finally of cerebral damage; and how ways of life and intrapersonal dynamics lead to the behavioral patterns that emerge. The table also attempts to show how somatic, interpersonal, and intrapersonal events are cyclically related.

Long-lasting disorientation and memory loss may develop at various rates, step-wise or insidiously, and they are often preceded by episodes of acute (reversible) organic mental syndrome. Episodes of this type may be related to malnutrition, as seems probable for some cases of the Wernicke-Korsakoff type. Also, infections, hypotension—as with myocardial infarction—surgical operations or accidents, and many other conditions may interfere with cerebral support.

The Psychiatric Reflection of the Aged Brain

Chronic brain syndrome refers to the irreversible state in which intellectual deficit is measurable repeatedly, with little evidence of learning or improvement. Some clinicians add that judgment is impaired, emotional lability may be present and troublesome, and insight into the condition on the part of the patient may be variable; these last are not helpful indices. With chronic brain syndrome there may also emerge disorders of mood, thought content, and behavior. These can be understood as reactions to the defects and as socially motivated attempts to minimize problems or to obtain aid. A marked alteration of mood, thought, and behavior does not signal severe brain damage; the reverse is closer to the truth. It is intellectual deficit—disorientation, memory loss, and deficiencies in general information and calculation—that comprise the syndrome, and it is these that can be relatively carefully measured by standardized techniques.

Etiology—general. To the psychiatrist it seems that the brain damage reflected by brain syndrome of the chronologically old is of multifactorial and variable etiology. There appear to be many sufficient causes for the damage, and they may occur in combination, reinforcing each other. No one of these causes need necessarily always be present.

Etiology—early influences. To begin with, brain cells may be lost on a genetic or gestational basis or because of problems in the delivery of the child; to this may be added losses in infancy or childhood, youth, and in late life. Among causes of such loss of cells may be accidents or illnesses of many kinds that directly or indirectly affect the brain: the effects upon physiology and metabolism of pollutants of air, food, or water, smoking, caloric excess, or the absence of essential nutrients. Even emergency emotion may play a part; it is known, for example, that with fear there may be hyperventilation which contributes to alkalosis; in the presence of marked CO_2 loss, cerebral circulation may be decreased by as much as one-half. Anything that may directly or indirectly affect brain nutrition, support, and metabolic processes may contribute to brain-cell losses. Eventually the ten billion or more cerebral cells are decreased to a critical level, not necessarily the same for all persons, at which point brain syndrome emerges.

Protections against psychiatric signs. The actual amount of cell loss at which deficits in mental functioning, as we now measure them, emerge differs from person to person. The difference seems to be related to such matters as the individual's education, occupation, and his habits of psychological, social, and emotional adaptation. Good psychological, social, and emotional habits may obscure the emergence of signs and a protective social setting may do the same.

If useful habits or ways of adaptation become well automatized, they mitigate the effects of the losses that come late in life. Nevertheless, with the loss of mentational resources there is usually a decrease in the ability of the individual to master what he should be able to deal with easily.

Heuristic Scheme of Pathodynamics

Table 2 shows schematically a sequence of events illustrating the many problems that may simultaneously be presented to physicians for solution. The scheme demonstrates that the therapist may be approached to help or may selectively choose to deal with a patient on one of many levels.

Certainly the treatment of psychiatric conditions related to the effects of aging upon the brain, as well as research bearing upon treatment, must take into consideration *the multiplicity of etiologic factors*—early and late—that are responsible for the loss of neurons reflected by brain syndrome; etiologic factors leading to brain damage are "causes" to be prevented, to be dealt with at their reversible points, or from whose direct or indirect effects the brain must be protected. But *the loss of resources* that results from mental impairment is also a cause for which compensatory devices can be supplied or taught, and which must lead the neuropsychiatrist to assay the patient's remaining assets and their optimal use. Moreover, *the environmental or intrapersonal challenges that decrease mastery* are "causes" that can be mitigated, evaded, or avoided. The decrease in mastery of social or personal demands can be regarded as causal.

Decrease in ability to work out means for the relief of tensions, whether biologically determined or of acquired type, and in obtaining gratifications leads to what the layman calls discomfort and frustration. This *helplessness* leads to a search for aid; the manner in which this search is conducted is usually, because of our modes of socialization, irrational, inefficient, and personally and socially disturbing. In addition, helplessness usually leads to *fear or anger*—to emergency emotion—which grossly influences how the search is elaborated and displayed. It is these reactions that are usually regarded as "the psychiatric illness" and the preceding events may mistakenly be disregarded.

TABLE 2
Components of Disorder: Psychodynamic Sequence

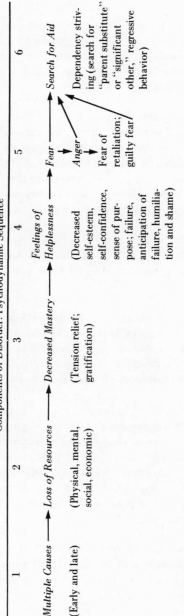

1	2	3	4	5	6
Multiple Causes →	*Loss of Resources* →	*Decreased Mastery* →	*Feelings of Helplessness* →	*Fear* → *Anger* →	*Search for Aid*
(Early and late)	(Physical, mental, social, economic)	(Tension relief; gratification)	(Decreased self-esteem, self-confidence, sense of purpose; failure, anticipation of failure, humiliation and shame)	Fear of retaliation; guilty fear	Dependency striving (search for "parent substitute" or "significant other," regressive behavior)

1. Multiple causes or initiating factors that occur either early in life and are reinforced or modified with aging, or occur late in life and are peculiar to old age, several of which may combine forces and some of which may be necessary but insufficient alone, result in

2. an absence or loss of resources for minimally adequate functioning, so that

3. there is decreased mastery of problems, challenges, and adjustments posed by internal changes (biologically determined drives or acquired needs), external changes and threats, with resulting

4. feelings of helplessness or actual powerlessness, and consequent

5. fear with accompanying or subsequent anger, with consequent

6. "rationally" or "irrationally" aimed and elaborated search for aid which becomes patterned in terms acceptable to the individual in terms of his personality organization based upon his past, his present, and his expectations; and contingent on his perception of what is acceptable to and likely to work in "his world," as well as by the social response it receives. In this search there are observable constellations of motivated personal action which range from apathy through pseudoanhedonia, display of helplessness, somatization, hypochondriasis, depression, and paranoid states to the most open and manipulative behavior. In predisposed persons there may be a physiologic shift to a new and relatively inefficient homeostatic level with depressive states, which are then revealed by altered appetite, bowel function, sleep, and other vegetative signs.

From Goldfarb, A.I. (Feb.) 1968. Clinical perspectives. *Psychiatric Research Report 23.* Reproduced with permission of American Psychiatric Association.

Patterns of Search for Aid

Provided the brain damage is not great enough to make patients stuporous, semicomatose, or vegetative, we may see a variety of patterns, alone or in combination. These patterns are reflections of the individual's search for understanding, reassurance, and emotional support—for attitudes of others that can help him quiet his fear and feelings of resentment, for attitudes that indicate he has a potential helper.

These patterns may be listed as follows: First, *apathy* is one way of searching for aid. If added to Alzheimer's disease—to organic mental syndrome—apathy may produce a vegetative organism in whom brain damage is still within the range that should permit the person to be ambulatory (Kahn and Goldfarb 1962). The person shows what Robert Kahn and I have called "excess disability." This is functional performance lower than the impairment would warrant. In the case of physical impairment, excess disability may be related to organic mental syndrome; in the case of mental impairment, excess disability may be part of the motivated search for aid.

Next is the pattern that can be termed *pseudoanhedonia*. The patient behaves and talks as though to say, "nothing can bother me any more, you can't hurt me, you can't please me, nothing matters."

Third is *somatization*. This may be the basis of an individual's preoccupation with complaints about the somatic concomitants of the emergency emotions, such as anginal pain or heaviness in the chest, or the aggravation, exploitation, or exacerbation of a physical disorder. With somatization we may see most clearly a blending and combining of the many factors—the causes, decrements in function, the effects on daily life and emotion—into a pattern of searching for aid.

Hypochondriasis should be listed next. Here the minor pain or harmless symptom or sign is seized upon as evidence of life-threatening disease or disorder. This symptom complex is a common precursor of clear-cut depression and may be present with a depressive reaction. Like apathy, somatization, and open display of helplessness, hypochondriasis is not only symbolic, justifying, and self-punitive, but it is punishing to the person who is being delegated parental status. In this sense all the patterns have a paranoid element.

In *depressive states*, a more clinically obvious disorder, other elements discussed here are always discernible. Hypochondriasis, a display of helplessness, and paranoid trends are commonly clearly present in depressive reactions. Relatively pure *paranoid states* are frequently seen when evidence of brain damage is minimal.

Exploitative-manipulative behavior may be the chief pattern with which aid is sought by older persons who have been dependent throughout life, or who in old age begin to show dependency in antisocial ways. Last, behavior maybe *coercive and punitive.*

These patterns may coexist, with one most obvious, or there may be a shift from one to another, contingent upon where the patient is, with whom he is dealing, how he is being responded to, and what he hopes for or expects. The symptoms usually cannot be considered as diagnostic of a particular disorder although we may classify them as if they were. They can usually be traced to the personality of the person before his mental impairment.

While it is clinically useful to regard each of these patterns as components of a constellation which may be variably displayed, it is nevertheless true that some people, because of their early experiences, display one or another of these components more obviously and frequently than any of the others. Genetic factors may, in some persons, contribute to the development of vegetative signs with depression or to paranoid states. In old age, previously unrecognized mood cyclic disorders may be "triggered" and emerge as more severe depressions than ever occurred earlier in the lifetime. Similarly, a propensity for schizophrenic reactions may be triggered by events of late life, the loss of resources, the decrements in mastery, and the consequent emotional state. Also to be kept in mind is the fact that a genetically determined propensity for mood cyclic or schizophreniform disorder constitutes a defect that interferes with mastery and leads to feelings of helplessness.

Prophylaxis, Treatment, and Care

All of this has been presented to emphasize that we can approach treatment, care, and prevention from the viewpoint of etiology, both early and late, by seeking assets to replace, substitute, or compensate for loss; by decreasing challenges to mastery; by dealing with the subjective state called helplessness; and by treating the emergency emotions and the behavior to which these lead.

The treatment of the patterns which phenomenologically emerge as "diseases," disorders, or reaction types may be understood as related to the preceding items in the sequence affecting individuals who differ genetically, experientially, and culturally. Direct approach to the early etiologic factors that influence and contribute to seriously impaired function is limited in the aged. This should be discussed, however, because it sheds light on prophylaxis. It is possible that if individuals are brought up and enculturated differently, now and in the future, there will be differences in aging and in the behavioral patterns displayed with aging. Deficiencies may be decreased in number or degree, and protective resources may be increased.

The loss of resources that often occurs with chronologic aging may lead to personal difficulties based on the absence or loss of resources occurring early. Whether Alzheimer's disease is of viral origin or genetically programmed and, like hypertension or diabetes, develops late in the lifetime, some causal factors may be necessary but not sufficient for the evolution of the syndrome. They may be joined during the individual's lifetime by events that reinforce or modify them. Many diseases are of multifactorial etiology. We must consider approaches that may modify not only the loss of brain cells, but that delay or minimize the emergence of brain syndrome in the presence of such loss. Attempts to encourage cell regeneration or revival by way of a ribonucleic-acid substance have not been successful; heparinization to improve circulation has not proved to be of value. Many other treatments, such as those of Bogomolets, Niehans, and Aslan, have not proved to be of value and may do harm.

Research in other methods and therapeutic agents continues and deserves attention. We have done studies, for example, of hyperbaric oxygen treatment (Jacobs et al. 1969) of organic mental syndrome, but have found it to be of no clinical usefulness. We concluded that, while it may be possible that hyperbaric oxygen treatment may be of benefit to selected groups, in our study this treatment did not benefit a randomly selected group of old persons with intellectual deficit of the type called organic mental syndrome.

What can be done about the loss of resources from late insults and developmental failures? Many commonly used prosthetic devices have proved helpful. When eyes fail, one uses glasses; when ears fail, one uses hearing aids; when a leg is missing, an artificial one or a crutch replaces it. When mentational resources fail, we may leave more time for tasks and convert the milieu so as to permit and encourage registration, recording, and recall. We can hang clocks and calendars on the wall, make personnel or help available to remind people of what to do and how to do it, and we can structure the day. For persons with a clinically measurable amount of so-called Alzheimer's disease or chronic brain syndrome, the milieu must be prosthetic. A protective setting can decrease the challenges to old and impaired persons; for example, providing transportation or making needed objects readily available is helpful. The milieu can be prosthetic and it can support the individual so that he can do the things he likes to do, but the environment can also be changed to decrease challenges and to supply the stimuli that bring pleasure.

In our society, a prosthetic milieu or protective environment connotes an institution. We would like, however, to make the outside world, the "community," more prosthetic and more supportive as well. This requires some social and cultural changes and warrants far more time for their exposition than is available here.

In late life the deficits reflected by brain-cell loss seem to be modified both by what has been learned and by the learning habits acquired early in life. What is usefully well-automatized is determined by many factors, beginning with the child-parent relationship, socioeconomic circumstances and opportunities, or lack of them in early life. People with good educational background, who have developed good habits of adjustment to many circumstances as well as good habits of self-orientation, will probably demonstrate fewer characteristics of brain syndrome than if they had been disadvantaged or deprived when they were young.

The early child-parent relationship is often determined by the socioeconomic status of parents. The education a child receives, the occupation he goes on to, the income he can earn is determined early, as is the establishment of the modes of psychological, emotional, and social adaptation that become his "way of life."

It is also important to remember that, in an individual with brain syndrome, behavior, mood, and content of thought vary greatly, contingent on his early life experience, training, and education. Failures in development or loss of resources during early life make mental impairment in old age more obvious. Psychological inhibitions developed in the child-parent relationship or its equivalent are the means of the enculturation of the child.

From diffuse energy and activity of the organism, inhibition molds and sculptures the adaptive personality of the child. The child learns to control impulses and to limit his behavior; he learns how to do things in a socially productive way, how to become socially integrative and relatively self-sufficient. We are most familiar with this process as it is said to affect psychosexual development. But there is more to psychological inhibition than sexual growth and development; how and what has been inhibited has much to do with how we assert ourselves in a variety of ways. In all of this are prophylactic implications that suggest the question: what kind of childhood promises the best old age in what kind of society?

Socialization tends, in most cultures, to decrease self-assertion. The individual whose self-assertion is greatly decreased is unable to utilize his resources to the fullest. Unable to say "pass the salt," he eats saltless steak. He may develop feelings of frustration, of not having what is needed or wanted, and then feel angry. With anger, however, he may be able to break out of his limited self-assertion and ask for what he should have been able to get had he not been restrained by excessive inhibitions taught him early in life.

Limitation of self-assertion is important in all areas, not merely in regard to sexual behavior. Psychodynamic psychiatry deals with events in the socialization of the child, how he became inhibited, what happened to his self-assertion, why he must become angry and aggressive and/or violent to achieve what he should be able to do constructively and easily.

Decrease in mastery. Individuals are daily, routinely concerned with the need to act in order to relieve tensions and to obtain gratifications. Not only must tensions of simple biologic origin be relieved, but so must the many tensions that arise from the enculturation process, like the need for relationship with other persons. Emotionally or psychologically determined needs for other people, as well as the way in which they are manifested, depend upon the manner of socialization. The need for a mate, a companion, friend, confidante, and what he is needed for, is very much related to how a person has been socialized, as is the need for admiration and praise for success in performance. Gratification of the desire to listen to music, to read, solve puzzles, use oneself adequately, is as real and urgent in old age as in former years. Some of these, like the need to solve puzzles or problems, are probably biologically determined, and they become inhibited in many individuals. Excessive inhibition of self-assertion and a decreased ability to utilize himself freely and fully deprive the person of the pleasure that comes from successful problem-solving through effective effector synthesis. The individual gives up easily, does not want to deal with challenges; he has been cheated of his biologic heritage.

As the individual grows old there is a decrease in his physical functional capacity, in his social and economic status; persons of real or fancied value are lost, and there may be loss of status and of role. Thus further losses are added to early acquired deficits and the capacity for mastery over everyday problems is decreased.

What can be done to increase the individual's capacity to master his environment? Keeping in mind the multiple causes for the elderly person's inability to marshall his resources provides clues to the variety of ways in which therapeutic leverage may be used to alleviate the patient's loss of mastery. We may add to his assets or redirect his use of them even when he is mentally impaired. Meticulous medical care previously mentioned as preventive must be mentioned again as being directly therapeutic. Old persons may need help with prostatism or cystocele and incontinence, with diarrhea, constipation, or obstipation of varying etiology.

Feelings of helplessness. For proper psychotherapeutic response we look upon the term "helplessness" as covering a wide spectrum. It includes a decreased sense of self-esteem, loss of confidence, and decreased ability to gain pleasure. When people cannot read or listen to music, are unable to visit or even talk with others, they feel they can no longer do things the way they used to and bring themselves no pleasure. They experience a decrease in sense of purpose; they have no quick and ready answer to the questions, "who am I, what am I, where am I going?" When pride is gone and feeling able to act is gone, and there is a loss of the capacity to provide onself with pleasures, then one is left without a sense of purpose. An actress who has lost her looks may say, "I have lost my identity." Much of what we call search for identity may be understood in these terms: a loss of purposivity caused by feelings of helplessness that follow upon loss of resources. These people feel that they are failures or they anticipate failure. Depending on the kind of culture they live in, these patients may also feel ashamed that they "can't do" and guilty of not fulfilling their obligations. There may be a sense of humiliation in not being able to "do what any man, any woman, any child could do." Irrationally these patients will embark upon a search for assistance which, as noted above, includes and is influenced by emergency emotion.

How can we deal with the complex, subjective experience called helplessness? This brings us once again to psychotherapy, to the need for understanding how individuals are enculturated in our society and how, in their distress, they irrationally search for aid. We need, first of all, to *recognize* their search and learn to help them believe they have found help.

Most people in our society are socialized to feel relatively secure and less helpless when they believe they have found and are maintaining a good relationship with selected types of other persons. When distressed by the loss of such persons or by the loss of resources to assure such relationships, they seek to replace the "significant other." The physician must permit the patient to feel he has gained the needed ally or friend, to feel dominant and assured that the person to whom he has turned for aid is dependable. This is the important role of the psychotherapist. He provides the figure or figures needed by the patient, either in himself or by way of nudging the individual toward a suitable person who will assume that role.

Psychiatrists, certainly, but all physicians and personnel who care for old persons should have training along these lines. All the helping professions need to learn that the best way to foster maximum self-sufficiency in old people is to let them become emotionally dependent and not to fear letting them become so. The old people will feel more protected, be less inefficiently symptomatic, and become more active as they feel in better control of their resources.

In responding to these needs, therapists are not "role-playing"; they simply do not refuse to let the patient believe he has found the person he needs and with whom he can feel secure. But we do not attempt to decrease the patterning of psychological inhibitions in older persons so as to yield a changed and reconstructed personality. This, at best, might take years of psychotherapeutic effort. As Rado said, "There is no point in trying to make our patients the healthiest people in the cemetery."

Psychiatric treatment of young persons often involves going back to inhibitions of self-assertion, as well as to the special and disorganizing needs they may have acquired. Young persons whom we help to deal with challenges effectively may once again become pleasure-providing, self-gratifying individuals. Even elderly persons who may have damaged brains can be helped to gain pleasure if they can be led to believe that they are effective and successful in personal relationships with those who care for them. While this is less than can be done with younger patients, it is actually as much as is done with most.

Feelings of fear and anger. There is an area for treatment, that of emergency emotions of fear and anger, which may respond to psychotherapy or which might be approached more effectively with pharmacologic agents. As Cannon and Rosenbleuth indicated many years ago, the emergency emotions should help to mobilize resources. If these emotions are intense, however, or if the organism is vulnerable to the effects of catecholamines deployed, as may be true for the old in whom homeostatic mechanisms are impaired, immobilization or disorganization may result. The aged person has limited cardiac and pulmonary function, limited musculoskeletal and cerebral-integration abilities, and emergency emotion may tend to harm his behavioral search for aid. With the advent of anger, the person may experience fear of retaliation and guilt. He may believe he should be punished for being "bad." This may require that the patient be allowed to feel he has encountered a mildly punitive but forgiving parental surrogate.

For the treatment of fear and anger, the emergency emotions, and the pathophysiologic states to which these lead, we have many psychotropic agents. The phenothiazines, for example, decrease fear and anger. Drugs of the phenothiazine type are useful in conditions in which catecholamine deployment has become deranged, and drugs of the tricyclic, anticholinergic type are helpful in treating so-called psychotic depressive symptomatology. Even in the old, barbiturates and similar medications have their place. Electroshock treatment is often useful.

The search for aid by the aged person, manifested by a variety of patterns that may accompany brain syndrome of mild to moderate degree, is a composite in which we have various processes to prevent, treat, or care for. It is best to recognize their totality and help whenever possible and expedient. To prevent symptoms by eliminating etiologic factors that are still operative, to give medical care as necessary for this purpose as well as to treat the organismal reaction, to provide prosthetic devices of all kinds including changes in social milieu or physical environment, and to add protective devices of all kinds is of importance. Basic to all this is response to the person's search for aid and treatment of his emergency emotion. This may mean such care as can be given only within a special "home" or institution where trained staff can be constantly responsive to the patient.

Summary

These factors have been presented in a schematic way to point to preventive as well as special treatment areas for research and development. Changes in socialization of the child and changes in our culture, including its values and the expectations it sets up, may help individuals to grow and develop optimally. To make old age less disturbed and less disturbing, attention to etiologic agents is obviously of greatest importance. With accidents, illness, intoxication, and the stress of emergency emotion, the brain of an old person may suffer from malsupport of a metabolic, nutritional, or vascular type; we have discussed some of the mechanisms involved. Drops in blood pressure, fever, infection, or electrolyte imbalance often result in acute brain syndrome. These insults may damage brain tissue irreversibly. Meticulous medical care, then, is an excellent preventive as well as treatment measure.

We are not now succeeding in delivering the type and quality of care implied by this schema to a great many persons with aged brains. In fact, at present, society seems to be organizing so as to block efforts to give good care to all persons with the kind of disorders we have described. There is a search for dramatically effective treatments, while what is well-known and useful seems neglected.

While we must continue to look for dramatically effective techniques, we must remember that we can now deliver very helpful services to old people with aged brains if we are willing to reorganize how and where we deliver comprehensive health care services. Because of its psychotherapeutic elements, whatever we offer old people along the lines of psychiatric, recreational, occupational, and special medical services now yields behavioral improvements, contributes to personal comfort, and should be well financed for delivery. We must capitalize on the aged person's readiness to feel less helpless and to derive pleasure from relationships with others by providing basic care—board, lodging, and basic medical care—in the most psychotherapeutic way. We must expand this by the addition of rational home care services for the people who can use them, while not denying rational and good institutional care to the very large group of people who must have it if their needs for care are to be answered.

References

Jacobs, E.A.; Winter, P.M.; Alvis, H.J.; and Small, S.M. 1969. Hyperoxygenation effect on cognitive functioning in the aged. *New Eng. J. Med.* 281:753.

Kahn, R.L., and Goldfarb, A.I. 1962. Criteria for the evaluation of "excess disability" in the aged and the quality of institutional care. Presented to fifteenth annual meeting of Gerontological Society, program abstract, p. 19.

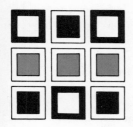

Psychopharmacological Aspects of Geriatric Medicine

H. E. Lehmann, M.D.

Douglas Hospital, Verdun, Quebec, Canada

Geriatric patients frequently develop psychiatric disorders, so frequently, in fact, that a new subspecialty of geriatric medicine has recently emerged which is becoming known as geropsychiatry. The psychiatric syndromes and symptoms observed in geriatric patients are not essentially different from those encountered in younger patients, but aging tends to develop certain "host qualities" in people which render them selectively more susceptible to certain stresses and more prone to certain pathological manifestations than to others. Because aging favors degenerative diseases, we see in geriatric patients a prevalence of psychopathology which is either the direct outcome of degenerative brain disease or reflects a functional reaction to it.

Thus we observe in many geriatric patients the signs and symptoms of the organic brain syndrome, mainly manifested in deficit symptoms such as confusion and loss of memory, emotional control, and intellectual power. While the acute organic brain syndrome is often reversible, the chronic organic brain syndrome usually leads to irreversible and progressive dementia.

But certain functional psychiatric symptoms are also frequently seen in geriatric patients, e.g., depression and paranoid delusions. These symptoms seem to be reactions to the human existential conditions of loss and threat of other losses, death, disability, economic insecurity, to which all geriatric patients are exposed. In addition to the prevailing condition of organic brain syndrome and the two functional syndromes of depressive and paranoid states, we also frequently observe alcoholism and dependence on sedative drugs as other typical forms of geriatric psychopathology.

It should be noted right away that the particular forms of senile amnesia, confusion, and dementia which characterize the organic brain syndrome are not natural and necessary consequences of aging – or a condition toward which all human life eventually moves. Although there is with advancing age a physiological diminution of memory and the aging individual's capacity to adjust to novel situations, these phenomena of normal senescence are essentially different and clearly distinguishable from the considerably more extreme pathological symptoms of, for instance, senile, presenile, or arteriosclerotic psychosis (Kral 1958; Overall and Gorham 1971).

The pathophysiology of organic brain disease is fairly well understood today, but we still know very little about the etiological factors leading to the development of senile psychosis or cerebral arteriosclerosis. We do not know what is responsible for the changes in colloidal structure, for the neuronal separation and deposition of amyloid in the brain parenchyma, what causes senile plaques to appear in senile dementia or vascular changes in cerebral arteriosclerosis.

General structural and metabolic changes in the aging brain are characterized by loss of neurons as well as by deterioration of cellular components and enzymatic activity. However, important factors behind these changes well may be, as Kety has pointed out, the normal progressive decline in oxygen utilization and blood supply in the CNS with advancing years (Kety 1956). It has been demonstrated convincingly that one of the most consistent physiological observations in all brain diseases is a substantial reduction of cerebral blood flow associated with increased circulatory resistance (Hedlund et al. 1964; Burke and Halko, quoted by Alvarez 1968).

However, although organic brain disease with its specific manifestations is particularly common in geriatric patients, we must not forget that there are also many geriatric patients who suffer from functional psychiatric disorders. A number of observers have demonstrated this from their own case material and have emphasized through many actual case histories that such functional psychiatric disorders in the aged—neuroses as well as psychoses—are often reversible and offer gratifying therapeutic possibilities. Unfortunately, we still see lamentably large numbers of geriatric patients who have been misdiagnosed as suffering from degenerative, progressive, organic psychoses, e.g., from senile psychosis. The presumption seems to be that a mentally disturbed person over 70 or 80 years of age could not possibly be suffering from anything else; as examples, the aged patient may manifest a depressive stupor, a manic excitement, a paranoid state, or a transient delirium, from all of which he could recover readily if given adequate medical treatment.

The aging organism's resistance to stress is reduced and thus certain therapeutic measures – e.g., the administration of certain drugs, which may produce comparatively harmless side effects in younger persons—may evoke dangerous reactions in older patients. Increased sensitivity to general anesthetics and narcotics in the aged has been reported as well as decreased sensitivity to the stimulant effects of amphetamines. The paradoxical response to barbiturates of many older persons is, of course, well known to the clinician.

By contrast, it is interesting that some pharmacological substances whose primary site of action is at the periphery, e.g., acetylcholine, histamine, and atropine, affect young and old persons in very similar ways.

Classification and Therapeutic Indications

Müller (1967) has attempted a classification of geriatric patients with psychiatric symptoms and their pharmacotherapeutic requirements on the basis of their electroencephalograms (EEGs). A first category contained patients with cerebral vascular insufficiency; their EEGs are characterized by slow waves, localized sharp and slow-wave abnormalities, or episodic slow-wave discharges in the left central-temporal region. He suggests that these patients receive drugs that increase cerebral blood supply. Müller's second category included patients with cerebral atrophy. Their EEGs are characterized by slowing and disappearing background activity which is later replaced by irregular slow waves and, terminally, by symmetrical slow-wave discharges. He feels that these patients might benefit from anabolic steroids. A third category contained patients with various types of functional psychopathology. Their EEGs are characterized by well-regulated alpha activity, low-voltage fast activity, or marked sharpness of the brain rhythms. For these patients — who represent the majority of geriatric patients requiring psychiatric treatment — he suggests treatment with neuroleptics, antidepressants, or anxiolytic drugs. So far, this interesting electrophysiologic classification has not been tested by giving this category of patients the proposed treatments.

A comprehensive review of pharmacotherapy in geropsychiatry has been presented by Lifschitz and Kline (1963). In another review I have divided pharmacotherapy of geropsychiatric patients into the following categories:

1. substitution or replacement therapy with various metabolic agents, vitamins, or hormones;
2. treatment with agents that influence cerebral circulation, i.e., mainly vasodilators and anticoagulants;
3. treatment with CNS stimulants or analeptics;
4. treatment with anxiolytic sedatives (minor tranquilizers);
5. treatment with neuroleptics (major tranquilizers);
6. treatment with antidepressants;
7. treatment with miscellaneous agents that have ranged from transplanted monkey glands, embryo cell injections (Niehans 1952), and royal bee jelly to Bogomolets' (1946) antireticular-endothelial serum and Aslan's (1956) procaine hydrochloride injections.

A Psychopharmacological Experiment

In the second part of this paper I want to report on an extended psychopharmacological experiment in geriatrics that we carried out at Douglas Hospital over more than six years (Lehmann and Ban 1970). The experiment was divided into two phases. Phase I was devoted to the development of a method for effective differentiation between our various geriatric patients. About one-half of our 300 geriatric patients had been in the hospital for many years; most of them were chronic schizophrenics who had grown old in the hospital. The other half were more recent admissions, and of those about one-half were suffering from organic brain syndromes. To differentiate between them we used four methods: (1) clinical diagnosis of the nosological entity to which each patient belonged; (2) psychopathology as determined by characteric symptom clusters, determined by a behavior rating scale; (3) performance on a battery of psychometric tests; and (4) changes in test performance following specific pharmacological loads.

Our experimental sample consisted of 107 geriatric patients who resided in the mental hospital. Their average age was 71 years. There were three diagnostic groups: (1) 38 patients suffering from organic brain disease, (2) 27 patients with paranoid schizophrenia, and (3) 42 patients with nonparanoid schizophrenia.

For the assessment of symptoms we used a modification of the Verdun Target Symptom Rating Scale (Lehmann and Ban 1970) which yielded five symptom clusters: (1) arousal, (2) affect, (3) mood, (4) mental integration, and (5) organicity.

Our psychometric test battery consisted of seven tests. Two tests were aimed at simple psychomotor functions: tapping speed and simple auditory reaction time. One test measured a perceptual (visual) function: critical flicker fusion frequency. Another test measured associational functions: word association time. Three tests evaluated attention and short-term memory: digits forward and backward, and a counting test requiring the patient to count up to a number at which he had been instructed to stop.

These tests, which we had used in a number of other investigations, have been described in several publications (Lehmann and Knight 1958; Lehmann 1959; Lehmann, Ban, and Kral 1968) and were evaluated for the purpose of this study in the following control and experimental groups: (1) a group of young (median age 20) healthy volunteers, (2) a group of aged (median age 72) healthy volunteers living at home, (3) a group of aged (median age 69) ambulatory patients attending a geriatric outpatients clinic, (4) a group of aged (median age 77) healthy volunteers living in an institution for the elderly, (5) a group of aged (median age 70) mental hospital patients suffering from functional psychoses, and (6) a group of aged (median age 71) mental hospital patients suffering from organic brain disease.

The pharmacological test loads consisted of:

1. a placebo — an intravenous injection of normal saline;
2. a psychostimulant — an intravenous injection of methamphetamine, 10 mg;
3. a CNS depressant — an intravenous injection of sodium amobarbital, 250 mg;

4. a cerebral vasodilator — a five-minute inhalation of a 5-percent carbon dioxide and 95-percent oxygen mixture.

Each subject was tested under each of the four pharmacological loads on four different days, separated from each other by at least one week.

The seven procedures of our psychometric test battery were administered to all subjects immediately before and 15 minutes after each pharmacological loading.

On our rating scales no significant differences appeared between symptom clusters in our three diagnostic groups, i.e., chronic brain syndrome, paranoid chronic schizophrenia, and nonparanoid chronic schizophrenia. This finding supports the clinical experience that it is often difficult to differentiate chronic, institutionalized patients suffering from functional psychoses from a similar group suffering from organic brain disease. Chronic psychotics frequently lose the specific clinical manifestations that were present in the acute stages, and diagnostic differences between various chronic psychiatric disorders become blurred.

By ranking the performance of our patients on the psychometric tests, however, we were able to discriminate between the functional and the organic disorders in patients.

Impairment of total performance in the efferent psychomotor tests (tapping speed and reaction time) was most pronounced in the patients with organic brain syndrome, while the nonparanoid schizophrenics showed the greatest decrement on the afferent perceptual test, i.e., critical flicker fusion frequency, and the paranoid schizophrenics in two central-cognitive tests, i.e., digits forward and backward.

We were surprised at the results of several of our pharmacological loadings. Neither the amphetamine nor the CO_2 loads produced statistically significant differences in test performance before and after the loads. Only with sodium amobarbital was a significant deterioration of test performance seen in all three diagnostic groups of patients as well as in the control groups.

Another interesting observation was that in a majority of the control group of young, healthy subjects the injections of saline, methamphetamine, and the inhalation of CO_2 all produced a slight (although not statistically significant) impairment of performance. In contrast to this observation, the majority of older patients suffering from organic brain disease *improved* their performance on the tests following these same pharmacological loads.

It is also interesting that, despite an overall statistically significant *impairment* of performance following sodium amobarbital by older and younger subjects combined, about 50 percent of our young controls (as well as 50 percent of the patients with organic brain diseases) *improved* their performance.

One possible explanation for some of these surprising observations is that the anxiety induced by the stress of the pharmacological load procedures affected the young subjects more than the aged patients, and the stress-induced anxiety in the younger controls was great enough to override the improvement that might have been produced by the administration of the stimulant (methamphetamine) or the cerebral vasodilator CO_2, while the same pharmacological effects might well have been responsible for greater improvement of performance in the less anxious older patients (Figure 1).

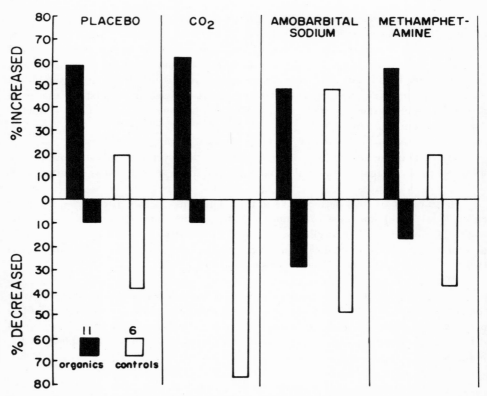

Figure 1. Relative percentages of geriatric brain-damaged patients and normal young controls showing tendency to improved (up) or impaired (down) performance on eight combined psychophysical tests immediately following treatment with four different agents.

The same mechanism might explain that the anxiolytic drug sodium amobarbital — although in general the most depressing pharmacological load in our study — improved the functioning of a higher proportion of our young control subjects than did any other load.

The second phase of our investigation — the therapeutic phase — involved 84 geriatric patients. All participants were treated over an eight- to twelve-week period with two or more drugs from a group of six different drugs we had chosen previously.

Before a patient was switched from one drug to another, a drug-free intermission of at least two weeks was imposed. Thirteen patients received all six drugs; 20 patients received five drugs; 8 patients were given three drugs; 8 patients got two drugs; and 19 patients received only one drug.

The following six drugs were administered in gradually increasing doses:

1. thioridazine — a neuroleptic phenothiazine, 75 to 150 mg daily;
2. meprobamate — an anxiolytic propanediol derivative, 600 to 1600 mg daily;
3. fluoxymesterone — a testosterone endocrine preparation, 5 to 20 mg daily;
4. nicotinic acid — a vasodilator vitamin, 300 to 3200 mg daily;
5. methylphenidate — a psychostimulant, 10 to 30 mg daily;
6. amitriptyline — a tricyclic antidepressant, 30 to 150 mg daily.

Psychiatric, psychometric, physical, and laboratory evaluations were done before each drug trial and then after four, eight, and twelve weeks. The psychiatric evaluation consisted of an interview and scoring on the Verdun Target Symptom Rating Scale, and the psychometric examination included our previously described test battery to which — during the treatment phase — we later added two other memory tests (picture recognition and paired associate learning).

Therapeutic Results

Our therapeutic results have been reported in greater detail in other publications. The following rank order of therapeutic efficacy emerged: thioridazine was most effective, producing improvement in three symptoms of our rating scale; then came nicotinic acid and fluoxymesterone with improvement in two symptoms each, followed by methylphenidate with improvement in one symptom; fourth was amitriptyline with improvement in one symptom as well as deterioration in another. Finally, meprobamate produced no significant improvement in this study but was associated with significant impairment in one symptom (Figure 2).

Table 1 presents the nature and magnitude of the clinical changes we observed with these drugs. Reduction of excitement and fatigue was responsible with thioridazine for improvement in the arousal parameter, while meprobamate *increased* fatigue in the doses administered, which might well have been too high for this age group. The affectivity parameter was favorably influenced by nicotinic acid and thioridazine which reduced anxiety, amitriptyline which decreased pathological autonomic reactions, and fluoxymesterone which reduced self-preoccupation; amitriptyline also lessened impulsiveness and thioridazine decreased suspiciousness. On the mood parameter, depression was reduced by thioridazine. Finally, on the mental integration parameter, methylphenidate decreased thought disorders, fluoxymesterone delusional thinking, and nicotinic acid perceptual disturbances. With amitriptyline there was impairment on this parameter, manifested by the more frequent occurrence of delusions in patients receiving this drug.

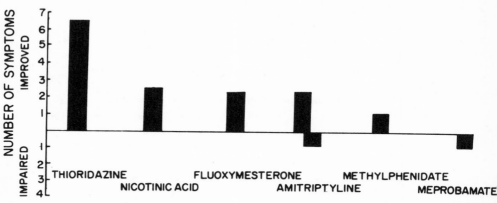

Figure 2. Number of rating scale symptoms on which statistically significant (positive or negative) therapeutic changes occurred with the six drugs.

Side Effects

A sharp rise in transaminase levels occurred in a few patients treated with fluoxymesterone; this rise was promptly reversed when the drug was discontinued, but in two patients it was high enough to call for discontinuation of the treatment.

Even low doses of amitriptyline not infrequently produced an aggravation of psychotic symptoms.

Meprobamate induced drowsiness and reduced spontaneous activity in some of our geriatric patients.

Changes in Test Performances

After twelve weeks of treatment with the different drugs, thioridazine and nicotinic acid produced a reduction of critical flicker fusion frequency, our measure of visual perception; meprobamate lead to improved performance on this test.

Meprobamate also was associated with increased tapping speed and improved performance on the digit-backward test.

Other drugs associated with improvement on memory tests were: methylphenidate (counting test) and fluoxymesterone (picture recognition and paired associate learning tests).

TABLE 1

		Amitriptyline	Fluoxymesterone	Meprobamate	Methylphenidate	Nicotinic Acid	Thioridazine
Mental Integration	Delusions	-0.02	+0.04				
	Thought Disorder				+0.03		
	Perceptual Disorders					+0.05	
Mood	Depression						+0.02
Affectivity	Preoccupation		+0.01				
	Impulsiveness	+0.05					
	Auton. Reactions	+0.05					+0.04
	Anxiety				+0.01		+0.04
	Suspiciousness						+0.05
Arousal	Fatigue		+0.001	-0.02			
	Excitement	+0.001					

Areas of clinical symptoms recorded on the rating scale on which statistically significant improvement occurred in the course of treatment. The direction of the change (+ or -) and the level of significance are indicated.

Possible Prediction of Therapeutic Drug Action

We were interested in the possible relevance of our observations for the prediction of the effects of particular drugs on particular patients. Tentatively we drew the following conclusions:

Thioridazine may be indicated for geriatric patients with symptoms of excitement, anxiety, high autonomic reactivity, increased fatigability, and suspiciousness;
nicotinic acid for anxious patients with perceptual disorders;
fluoxymesterone for delusional patients who are preoccupied with their body functions;
methylphenidate for patients with thought disorders who are not anxious or delusional.

Amitryptiline and meprobamate were of no particular therapeutic value in our sample of hospitalized geriatric patients with psychotic symptoms.

One of our hypotheses had been that changes in psychometric test performance immediately following the pharmacological loads would be related to the long-term therapeutic effects of certain drugs. Our statistical analysis did not support this hypothesis since no statistically significant correlations emerged. Our clinical impressions, however, based on our observations of patients and corresponding inspection of the experimental data, seemed to point to certain predictive relationships. In brief, our data suggest:

1. a favorable therapeutic result for thioridazine in patients who show a decrease of test performance following pharmacological loads of CO_2 or methamphetamine;
2. a favorable response to fluoxymesterone in patients showing improved test performance following loadings with CO_2 and methamphetamine, but impaired test performance following amobarbital;
3. a favorable response to nicotinic acid in patients who show improved test performance following CO_2 inhalation, but respond with impaired test performance to the administration of methamphetamine and amobarbital;
4. patients who perform worse on the tests following CO_2 inhalation might respond well to methylphenidate (Table 2).

None of these observations and impressions are based on hard experimental evidence since our drug trials were not done under double-blind conditions or with placebo controls, and we could not be sure that the quantitative results which were statistically significant had not occurred by chance. However, if our hunches can be confirmed it would in future be possible to select a specific drug that would be best suited for the treatment of psychiatric symptoms in a given geriatric patient, not only on the basis of empirical trial and error but on the basis of certain clinical characteristics and

TABLE 2

Relationship Between Overall Psychometric Performance Change
After Pharmacologic Loads and Therapeutic Response

Drug	Therapeutic Responses	Carbon Dioxide	Methamphetamine	Na Amobarbital
Amitriptyline	−		−	
Fluoxymesterone	+	+	+	−
Meprobamate	±	±		
Methylphenidate	+	−		
Nicotinic Acid	+	+	−	−
Thioridazine	+	−		−

+ indicates improved test performance or favorable therapeutic response.
− indicates impaired test performance or unfavorable therapeutic response.

experimental findings.

Eventually the pharmacological load procedure could probably be considerably simplified. For instance, our data suggest that the direction of response changes in the performance of a few simple tests following a five-minute inhalation of a 5-percent CO_2 – 95-percent O_2 mixture might give important clues for the selection of special drugs to be used for therapy. As an example, patients who improve their test performance after CO_2 inhalation will probably respond best to fluoxymesterone and nicotinic acid, and patients whose test performance becomes worse following CO_2 might respond better to methylphenidate and thioridazine. Since brief inhalation of a 5-percent CO_2 – 95-percent O_2 mixture involves no particular hardship or risk for geriatric patients, but may even have a therapeutic effect by itself, this simple procedure might well deserve wider application.

Other Recent Findings in Geropsychiatric Pharmacotherapy

Our previous studies had revealed that thioridazine, nicotinic acid, and fluoxymesterone were the three most effective drugs of the six we had tried. In a follow-up investigation we reevaluated the effects of these three drugs given singly, and also studied the various combinations of two of these best drugs and of all three combined, in a placebo-controlled clinical trial in similar groups of chronic hospitalized geropsychiatric patients. One important finding was that during twelve weeks of placebo administration we observed a statistically significant deterioration in several symptoms, i.e., mannerisms and posturing, hallucinations, uncooperativeness, and perceptual disturbances, suggesting strongly that placebo administration is insufficient to arrest or improve geropsychiatric pathology.

Furthermore, the combination of all three drugs, i.e., thioridazine, nicotinic acid, and fluoxymesterone, did not produce any improvement. On the contrary, significant behavioral deterioration occurred with this treatment regime in three symptoms of our rating scale. Finally, this triple-drug combination induced many adverse side effects, some of which were quite serious.

With high doses of nicotinic acid alone (3,000 mg) we observed increased anxiety and a total of 49 adverse reactions. Thus, a combination of the three most effective drugs or high doses of nicotinic acid alone seem to be contraindicated in the treatment of chronic geropsychiatric patients.

Fluoxymesterone alone maintained the patients without improvement or deterioration of behavior, but 40 different adverse reactions were observed with this treatment, and eight patients had to be taken off the drug because of pathological laboratory findings in liver-function tests.

Thioridazine alone produced improvement in one symptom but deterioration in three other symptoms. It was also associated with numerous, though mild, side effects.

The most favorable effects were observed in those patients who received a mixture of fluoxymesterone plus thioridazine or fluoxymesterone plus nicotinic acid. None of the patients receiving these drug combinations had to be taken off the trial because of adverse side effects. The best therapeutic results and the fewest side effects were observed with the combination of fluoxymesterone plus thioridazine at a dosage of 75 mg of thioridazine and 10 mg of fluoxymesterone daily over a period of twelve weeks.

Our results suggest that pharmacotherapy seems to hold promise in the clinical management of geropsychiatric problems and that the most successful treatment may be found in the combined application of various pharmacological approaches. The recent literature abounds with reports of a great variety of drugs proposed for different geropsychiatric problems.

Pentylenetetrazol, in a double-blind controlled study by LaBrecque and Goldberg (1967) improved appearance of geriatric patients in 48 percent, memory in 38 percent, and working capacity in 25 percent. Similar results were reported by Levy (1963) and even better results by Deitrick (1967) who combined the drug with nicotinic acid. In a more recent study by Leckman et al. (1971), pentylenetetrazol produced improvement in the symptom areas of unusual thought content, irritability, consciousness alteration, and autonomic reactivity; a trend toward improvement of memory was also observed. At the same time a control group receiving placebo showed significant deterioration in the symptom areas of grandiosity, self-preoccupation, and consciousness alteration. The authors noted that nine of their ten patients on the active drug lost weight.

Schindler, Steininger, and Waitusch (1968) reported that, with the drug noveril, out of 100 geropsychiatric patients presenting mainly with affective symptoms, 60 percent showed very good and another 12 percent slight improvement. Particularly favorable effects were noted in hypochondriacal complaints. This substance has some analgesic action.

Surprising improvement was reported by Chynoweth and Foley (1969) with high doses of corticoid steroids in patients suffering from presenile dementia — a condition which until now has been refractory to all treatment. The authors feel that the presenile dementias belong to the group of collagen diseases and that autoimmune factors may play a role in their etiology.

Centrophenoxine, possibly a precursor of cerebral acetylcholine, has been studied by several European workers who noted that the drug has psychoanaleptic effects in geropsychiatric patients suffering from various organic brain syndromes. The drug is reported to increase drive and improve mood and has also been recommended specifically for the treatment of confusional states such as are seen, for instance, in delirium tremens. Experiments have demonstrated that centrophenoxine allows brain tissue to function better under hypoxic conditions and reduces the amount of the age-related pigment lipofuscin in most parts of the central nervous system of senile guinea pigs (Gerstenbrand, Hoff, and Prosenz 1963; Espie 1966; Wietek 1966; von Bergener 1967). Negative results with the drug in the treatment for senile dementia were reported by Bower and McDonald (1966).

Lipotropic enzymes have been tried in the treatment for arteriosclerotic dementia by Hall and Harcup (1969). They treated 49 patients with Vasolastine, a mixture of citrogenase, aminoacid oxidase, and tyrosinase complexes. The authors observed statistically significant improvement in subjective complaints of depression and lack of energy, but other beneficial effects did not reach significance. Other attempts to treat atheroma of the CNS with enzymes have included the administration of B-glucuronidase (Kayatan 1960), cytochrome C (Altschul 1959), and hepatic catalase (Hunter 1960).

In dealing with the cerebrovascular insufficiency which prevails in many geropsychiatric conditions, favorable effects have been reported with the drug cyclandelate. It could be demonstrated that the drug improves cerebral blood flow, has a beneficial effect on the EEG, and improves reaction time, mental functions, and behavior (Stöker et al. 1971). The vasodilator drug papaverine also was found in one double-blind study of 30 geriatric patients to be more effective than placebo in relieving thirteen of fifteen target symptoms related to chronic brain syndromes. Favorable effects were observed on depression, excitability, insomnia, somatic complaints, restlessness, apathy, and withdrawal. There were numerous mild side effects (Stern 1970).

Fünfgeld (1970) has shown that in some cases normal oxygen uptake in brain tissue may be associated with selective disturbance of glucose utilization, which may be reduced. He treated 86 patients suffering from chronic diffuse cerebral vascular and metabolic processes with Actihaemyl (known in Switzerland and Austria as Solcoseryl), which is a protein-free extract obtained from the blood of young calves. Its influence on cerebral metabolism is not entirely clear, but of the patients treated with this drug intravenously from two to four weeks, 57 percent showed good or very good improvement, and there were no toxic symptoms. The same author reported that he treated 200 patients with pyritinol (Encephabol) administered orally. Fifty-two percent of his patients showed very good improvement with this drug, and in the EEGs there was a tendency to faster frequencies and higher amplitudes after treatment. Pyritinol reduces glucose in arterial and venous blood, but leads to increased cerebral glucose uptake and utilization in animals and human beings after ten to fourteen days. Adrenaline-induced lipolysis is reduced by the drug. Finally, Fünfgeld found that vitamin B_{12} had a favorable influence on drive and initiative in more than 100 patients.

Fünfgeld concludes that slowly developing organic brain syndromes after 55 years of age, as well as paranoid hallucinatory psychosis, can be favorably influenced by pharmacotherapy; however, little success can be obtained with rapidly progressive cerebral atrophy such as occurs in Pick's and Alzheimer's disease.

Summary

Psychiatric symptoms in geriatric patients may be of organic or functional origin. The causes of degenerative brain diseases affecting the brain parenchyma or its vascular structure and producing the so-called organic brain syndrome, are still unknown. Functional psychiatric disorders in the aged are often characterized by depressive or paranoid symptoms and may represent reactions to the old person's existential condition of increased inner and outer threats and losses. These functional psychiatric disorders in the older person often respond to tranquilizers, neuroleptics, and antidepressants as well as they do in younger patients. Chronic organic brain syndromes, however, respond only partially to these drugs. Experimental new approaches attempt to combat the underlying metabolic pathophysiology of the organic brain syndrome and aim at increasing cerebral blood flow, improving oxygen and glucose uptake of cerebral tissue, and at substitution of hormone and enzyme deficiencies. So far these attempts have achieved only limited success.

A systematic therapeutic trial with a variety of drugs revealed that a combination of thioridazine and fluoxymesterone, given daily over a twelve-week period, produced the best therapeutic results in a group of hospitalized, chronic geropsychiatric patients. The same clinical trial demonstrated that it might eventually be possible to obtain predictors for a geropsychiatric patient's response to a particular drug by observing changes in his responses to simple tests after the administration of pharmacological "loads," e.g., the brief inhalation of 5-percent CO_2 − 95-percent O_2 mixture.

References

Ahmed, A. 1968. Thioridazine in the management of geriatric patients. *J. Amer. Geriat.* 16(8):945.
Altschul, R. 1959. Einfluss von Cytochrome C auf Serum Cholesterin. *Kreislaufforsch.* 48:844.

Aslan, A. 1956. A new method for prophylaxis and treatment of aging with novocain-eutrophic and rejuvenating effects. *Therapiewoche* 7:14.

Assessment in Cerebrovascular Insufficiency. An International Symposium on Various Methods of Assessing the Effects of Cyclandelate on Higher Cortical Function, Würzburg 1970. G. Stöker, R.A. Kuhn, P. Hall, G. Becker, E. van der Veen (eds.). Stuttgart:Georg Thieme Verlag, 1971.

Bergener, von M. 1967. Behandlung psychiatrischer Krankheitszustände in Alter. *Hippokrates* 38:432.

Bogomolets, A.P. 1946. *The Prolongation of Life*. New York:Duell, Sloan & Pearce.

Bower, H.M., and McDonald, C. 1966. A controlled trial of A.N.P. 235 ("Lucidril") in senile dementia. *Med. J. Aust*. 2(6):270.

Burke, G., and Halko, A. 1968. Quoted in editorial by W.C. Alvarez. *Geriatrics* 23:96.

Chynoweth, R., and Foley, J. 1969. Pre-senile dementia responding to steroid therapy. *Brit. J. Psychiat*. 115:703.

Deitrick, R.A. 1967. Pentylenetetrazol with nicotinic acid in the management of chronic brain syndrome. *J. Amer. Geriat*. 15:191.

Espie, M.J. 1966. Pharmacologie de la centrophénoxine. Application au delirium tremens. *Lyon Med*. 215:935.

Fünfgeld, E.W. 1970. Ergebnisse medikamentöser Therapie bei älteren Patienten mit cerebralorganischen Störungen. *Nervenarzt* 41:352.

Gerstenbrand, F.; Hoff, H.; and Prosenz, P. 1963. Therapeutische Erfahrungen mit Lucidril bei neuro-psychiatrischen Krankheitsbildern. (Therapeutic experiences with Lucidril in neuropsychiatric disease pictures.) *Wien. Med. Wschr*. 113(25-26):539.

Hall, P. and Harcup, M. 1969 suppl. A trial of lipotropic enzymes in atheromatous ("arteriosclerotic") dementia. *Angiology* 20:287.

Hedlund, S.; Köhler, V.; Nylin, G.P.; Olsson, R.; Regnström, O.; Rothström, E.; and Åström, K.E. 1964. Cerebral blood circulation in dementia. *Acta Psychiat. Scand*. 40:77.

Hunter, J.D. 1960. Nicotinic acid therapy in patients with coronary disease. *New Zeal. M.J*. 59:60.

Kayatan, S. 1960. Atherosclerosis and betaglucuronidase. *Lancet* 2:667.

Kety, S.S. 1956. Human cerebral blood flow oxygen consumption as related to aging. In *The Neurologic and Psychiatric Aspects of the Disorders of Aging*. Baltimore:Williams & Wilkins.

Kral, V.A. 1958. Senescent memory decline and senile amnestic syndrome. *Amer. J. Psychiat*. 115:361.

LaBrecque, D.C., and Goldberg, R.I. 1967. A double blind study of pentylenetetrazol combined with niacin in senile patients. *Curr. Ther. Res*. 9:611.

Leckman, J.; Ananth, J.V.; Ban, T.A.; and Lehmann, H.E. 1971. Pentylenetetrazol in the treatment of geriatric patients with disturbed memory function. *J. Clin. Pharmacol*. 11(4):301.

Lehmann, H.E. 1959. Methods of evaluation of drug effects on the human central nervous system. In *The Effect of Pharmacologic Agents on the Nervous System*. Baltimore: Williams & Wilkins.

Lehmann, H.E., and Ban, T.A. 1970. Pharmacological load tests as predictors of pharmacotherapeutic response in geriatric patients. In *Psychopharmacology and the Individual Patient*. J.R. Wittenborn, S.G. Goldberg, and P.R.A. May (eds.). New York:Raven Press.

Lehmann, H.E.; Ban, T.A.; and Kral, V.A. 1968. Psychological tests: Practice effect in geriatric patients. *Geriatrics* 23:160.

Lehmann, H.E., and Knight, D.A. 1958. Psychophysiological testing with a new phrenotropic drug. In *Trifluoperazine: Clinical and Pharmacological Aspects*. H. Brill (ed.). Philadelphia:Lea & Febiger.

Levy, S. 1963. Pharmacological treatment of aged patients in a state mental hospital. *JAMA* 153:1260.

Lifschitz, K., and Kline, N. 1963. Psychopharmacology of the aged. In *Clinical Principles and Drugs in the Aging*. J. Freeman (ed.). Springfield:Charles C Thomas.

Müller, H. 1967. Drugs — EEG and the aged. Presented at a symposium on Psychoactive Drugs in the Aged. Quebec Psychopharmacological Research Association, Quebec, Canada.

Niehans, P. 1952. Zur Geschichte der Zellular-Therapie, zugleich eine Richtigstellung. *Hippokrates* 27:219.

Overall J.E., and Gorham D.R. Feb. 1971. Organicity versus old age in objective and projective test performance. *Psychometric Laboratory Reports* No. 16. Dept. of Neurology and Psychiatry, Psychometric Laboratory. The University of Texas Medical Branch, Galveston, Texas.

Schindler, Von R.; Steininger, E.; and Waitusch, A. 1968. Noverilbehandlung von psychiatrischen Alterpatienten. *Wien. Med. Wschr.* 118:368.

Silver, D.; Debow, S.L.; Lehmann, H.E.; Kral, V.A.; and Ban, T.A. Nov. 1967. The comparative effectiveness of psychoactive drugs in hospitalized geriatric patients. Presented at the Quebec Psychopharmacological Research Association Meeting, Quebec, Canada.

Stern, F.H. 1970. Management of chronic brain syndrome secondary to cerebral arteriosclerosis, with special reference to papaverine hydrochloride. *J. Amer. Geriat.* 18(6):507.

Stöker, G. 1971. Cerebral functions and cerebral blood flow. In *Assessment in Cerebrovascular Insufficiency* by G. Stöker, R.A. Kuhn, P. Hall, G. Becker, and E. van der Veen. Stuttgart: Georg Thieme Verlag.

Wietec, H.F. 1966. Zum Einfluss von Centrophenoxin auf das Alterspigment Lipofuscin in Nervenzellen. (The influence of centrophenoxine on lipofuscin, the pigment of old age in nerve cells). *Arzneimittel-Forschung* 16(8):1123.

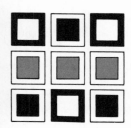

Some Psychodynamic Aspects of Agedness

Jack Weinberg, M.D.

Illinois State Psychiatric Institute and
Abraham Lincoln School of Medicine
University of Illinois, Chicago, Illinois

My assignment is to discuss some psychodynamic aspects of what I like to call agedness rather than aging. Aging is an ongoing process difficult of assessment. Agedness, however, is an assumed stance on the part of the organism that may or may not be due to organ dysfunction but may be behavioristically characteristic of a unified system complex of roles, assigned, ascribed, and much too often acquired. It may be both character and pathology. It may be independent of any overt manifestation of organic disease and thus present itself as a mode of coping or adaptive behavior most economical to the character structure of the individual. One may manifest agedness quite early in one's life, behavioristically speaking. Thus it is the manifest behavior of the individual that interests me and the latent meaning of its content that intrigues me. For it is the understanding of the behavior and not only its origin that can produce the proper responses in dealing with it and with the problems that may ensue.

Many clinicians tend to reify the names of abnormal psychological conditions and thus assume their reality as entities. A more consistent clinical view would, to my mind, regard diagnoses as names given to sets of extreme variations of different kinds of behavior. The behavioral modalities subsumed under a diagnostic category are not describable as unitary. It is not the diagnoses that have a reality reference but rather the behavioral variation the diagnoses describe. In any type or class of behavior one will see extremes, and the laws that govern and describe those extremes also govern and describe the nonpathological functioning. Thus the idea of the continuity between normal and abnormal can be established and have a meaning.

Furthermore, it may be an arguable fact, but fact nevertheless, that no one behavior is unique to a diagnostic category. Individual symptoms, therefore, are not reliable indices of a psychopathological grouping. When precise and definite etiological factors have been

209

isolated and the pathogenesis is well understood, the disease entity itself may certainly be used to define a target population. However, most studies on the psychopathological conditions of aging (and I may say other groupings) do not define etiological or pathogenic factors and, lacking such focus, lead many of us to what may be described as empirical conclusion on behavioral patterns.

As an example, this state of affairs has led investigators to two general approaches to perception-psychopathology relationships. One approach regards perception as an independent variable and directs our attention to the effects of disordered perception on personality development and consequent behavior. Another regards psychopathological conditions as independent variables and regards the perceptual behavior as outcomes or effects. I, for one, an adherent to the latter notion, have long since postulated the exclusion of stimuli in later life as an outcome or effect of a psychopathological if not psychodynamic condition. Perception refers to a perceptual act that transforms a physical stimulus into psychological information. This transformation involves complex processes including reception of the stimulus, registration, the processing of the registered information, and the checking of the information against continued input. Eventually the organismal organization is meant to interpret all of the above in the light of its life experiences and effect action. Sensory cognitive, conceptual, affective, and motor processes all are linked with each other in any given perceptual act. Most psychiatrists have long since recognized the crucial significance of perception, its central role in the development of those modulatory and controlling structures Freud has designated as the ego or, as I like to call it, the problem-solving self. For the perceptual act reflects the psychological point of contact between a person and his internal and external milieu. Its principal function is to convey information from his environment for integration with other psychological functioning such as memory, judgment, and anticipation. Obviously it also receives and carries information about the nature and consequence of the perceiver's actions. Perception is thus a central ingredient in effective adaptation, in the fitting-in process between the individual and his environment.

As the individual develops and moves towards active mastery he can no longer depend on the instrumentality of others as in infancy, childhood, and adolescence, but must amplify and coordinate the executive potential of his own body parts, which cease to be independent information and pleasure receptors, and take up their collaborative, productive functions. In later life, due to intrinsic and extrinsic vectors, recapitulation of early developmental sequences may take place, moving the individual from productivity to receptivity and, in effect, to dependence on the mastery or the instrumentality of others, an adaptive approach which, in the belief of some, is characterized by gross coercive dependence and/or by the disruption of proper ego functioning.

The threat of organic deficits or destruction within, plus the welling-up of heretofore unacceptable but controlled impulses, and the all too frequent deterioration of the individual's socioeconomic status tax the adaptive capacities of the ego to the utmost. To master the threat of dissolution of its boundaries and to ward off any break with reality, the aging organism — having at its disposal a lowered psychic energy supply and being unable to deal with all stimuli — begins to exclude them from awareness. While, of course, the nature of the receiving organ obviously influences reception, it has been carefully pointed out that perception is not a passive process. The physical stimulus is organized and transformed at the point of reception, and I like to believe that it never goes beyond the point of the sensory receptor.

The infant, too, is faced by the problem of too many stimuli and little ego development to help him cope with them. The very young, however, can and do take refuge in sleep or withdrawal to allow a gradual exposure to the clamor and the slow, measured, developmental integration of stimuli and the evolvement of acceptable responses to them. Then, too, the very young are helped by supportive figures who are ever ready to supply ego judgment and strength to the struggling new organism. None of these elements is available, nor is it acceptable to the aging individual; hence the exclusion.

Though it may be argued by some that the mechanism of exclusion of stimuli is identical to the familiar mechanism of denial, it is my belief that this defense is rather different. Denial, in my view, implies that a stimulus has been received, cathechticized, invested in, and then cathexis is withdrawn. Not so with the exclusion of stimuli. A stimulus may be blocked at the point of entry by a threshold lowered only for those stimuli relevant to one's narcissism — by which, at this point, I mean survival value. The problem as I continue to see it is how to assess the rate and extent of the exclusion experimentally so as to utilize this mechanism as a psychobiological measure of aging.

Based on the above assumptions and the assumption that our society is neglectful, if not hostile, to the needs of the aged, I have allowed myself psychodynamic formulation on some aspects of their behavior.

The sensory organs envelop each individual with personal spatial boundaries, boundaries within which messages may be perceived, and which may differ in dimensions and scope for each organ. Tactile language would therefore be the closest and, unless invited or eagerly yearned for, may be the most encroaching and threatening of all stimuli received. Thermal, olfactory, aural, and visual stimuli, in that order, provide ever-increasing spatial territoriality for meaningful messages of increasing complexity to reach the human being, for him to decode, and to give the proper response. Each of these personal spaces may have a "do not trespass" sign, not discernible to others but quite well delineated for the comfort of each organism.

When cultural determinants are added to these biologically determined boundaries, the problem becomes even more complex. Unless invited, encroachment on one's personal space becomes an invasion of one's privacy. Cultural values, biases, and practices tend to decrease the allowable areas of intrusion, inhibit the sending out and receiving of messages, and thus further thwart the language of communication. The transactional reciprocity between the human organism and its circumambience is a thing of beauty to behold. For, ironically enough, as visual and auditory acuity diminish and the environment language becomes less discernible, the aged themselves join the vast throngs of the invisible and untouchable in our society.

It isn't that I am unaware of the effects of organic deficits. My emphasis is on the effects of one's inner perception of the self and one's ambience, and their effects on sensory organ functioning. While all may agree with what is here stated, the tendency is to arrive at quick closure on the effects of the first, and a more comprehensive therapeutic effort may be sacrificed on the altar of organicity. Thus, in a recent paper concerning the needs of the elderly for tactile relationships, of the need for intimacy and touch, I wrote, "The sensory organ of the aged person's skin often becomes dull, as if in response to an anticipated deprivation. There is no need to feel, if feelings are to be denied." And again: "Visually the older person is more concerned with messages in his environment dealing with movement. Available data suggest that he relies more heavily on visual information channeled through the periphery of the eye, which magnifies movement, than on information received by means of detailed and clear vision. Psychologically it is as if the older person anticipates some external threat to his being and is alert to ward off an offending object, or in search of a supportive figure."

Complicating matters even more is the fact that the behavioral patterns as manifested by the aged are bound to inner secret legends each person has about himself. As psychiatrists we are engaged in a type of life review of each one of our patients. The life review allows us to perceive the life style or more often the life theme, as Binswanger calls it, of the individual. The life theme of a person, as an example, may be of emptiness and a constant search for the filling of the self, as one may encounter in a depressed individual. What is not so apparent, even to an astute observer, is the personal legend, as I like to call it, that pervades our being and motivates our behavior. I use the term legend, for in all of us the concept of the self as a dynamic force, interacting with the environment, is more often than not tinged with wish rather than reality and is thus distorted and obscured. When the legend of the self is not in concert with the facts as they are, discomfort and disease make their appearance. The legend leads to a romanticizing of the self and a poetic interpretation of reality, which arouses skepticism and even hostility toward the holder of the dream. There are personal realities, therefore, that transcend the obvious truth.

To move on to another dimension, man recognizes that the existing harmony and interrelationships in the world about him and within him bespeak an interdependence between them. The loss of any of the components or systems calls for a new adaptation and adjustment to the whole. The observation of these phenomena added to man's own life experiences from infancy to maturation in a complex society make it quite apparent to him that he cannot exist isolated from other interacting individuals. He can manage to do so for a given period of time, particularly when there is hope that the isolation will eventually end. He cannot manage, though, if the isolation is not self-imposed or if there is no hope of its amelioration. This, however, is precisely the situation faced in later life within our culture. The gradual isolation of the aging organism into a state of aloneness is the great tragedy of aging.

I use the term aloneness because it is descriptive of the intensely experienced inner affect related to the gradual isolation that takes place and is a physical or geographic state. Aloneness, of course, is a result of a number of factors. A very real one is the dispersal and death of friends and members of the family. Each loss necessitates a rearrangement of the equilibrium the individual had set up for comfortable functioning. Each loss, too, releases energy previously invested but which now needs a new object. The aging person searches for a substitute but there are no takers. There is no replacement of family and there are no bidders for his friendship. When the aging individual attempts to reestablish equilibrium by attempting to reinvest the freed libido in new objects in the environment, he meets a wall of resistance. Having no place to go, this freed energy is turned inward, and it is either reinvested in organs or organ systems and appears in the guise of somatic complaints, or it is experienced as pain and ruminatory recapitulation of a past life experience. The aged then appear to be egocentric, selfish, and preoccupied with inner rumblings of the self.

Within the final span of years the aged must also face the twin spectrum of physiological losses and eventual death, of which the above are but a part. Losses may be handled by denial, overcompensatory mechanisms, or projection. Grief may be a constant companion which takes on the appearance of depression. Equally common is the method of dealing with losses, and the one most troublesome to respond to is that of projection. It is most often expressed by complaints of the aged that someone is cheating or lying to them, stealing or taking things away from them. It is a rebuke and an expression of anger at the fact that internal biological losses are being sustained, that mastery over hitherto controlled functions and impulses is threatened, and influence over one's family and environment wanes. The "thieves, robbers, and cheats" are usually members of the family, friends, relatives, and caretakers who can least comprehend the accusations made against them, and who in turn respond in anger which results in mutual frustration, distrust, and alienation.

Psychodynamically the above is quite clear. By taking over functions for the aged, we do rob them of mastery and control. While it may be necessary as a protective device and to save the aged from their own judgmental deficits, the fact that control of their independent actions is being usurped cannot be denied. The response on the part of the aged is either that of rage or accusation, hanging on to any vestige of control, or by denial that may be either vigorous or pitiful, depending on the circumstances. Frequently the aged will begin to hold on and cling to many seemingly meaningless objects. Hoarding is not uncommon, whether it be of food, priceless objects, or trifles. This, too, needs to be understood in the light of ever-increasing losses. The more often the aged person loses close friends — others with whom he has shared life experiences — the greater is his need to hold on to inanimate objects with which he has shared common experiences. These objects replace and are substitutes for cherished reunions and memories when very few, if any, friends are left to meet with and reminisce. Chaotic disorder to the observer may represent organizing strength to the observed old person, so that forbearance should be the guiding rule.

Cultural patterns, too, play a great role in determining variables in human behavior. These include not only moral standards and mores but also more subtle patterns of motivation and interpersonal relationships. Variations in judgment and systems of belief, like religion and philosophies, have been integrated with other cultural patterns, like child-rearing practices, by the cultural anthropologists. As a result of this synthesis, there is now clearer understanding of the effects of one or the other on the individual and on the cultural patterns he has developed. The values the child accepts, introjects, and incorporates into himself have much to do with defining his attitude toward aging people and later toward himself as an aging person. If in our society the aged are perceived as unattractive, unproductive, old-fashioned, useless, querulous, etc., then we in our youth absorb these concepts, make them part of ourselves, and apply them to ourselves in later life. Clearly a built-in system of self-depreciation or denial and dynamic processes determine behavior.

We need, therefore, to examine some specifics of our culture, its value system, and their continued effects on behavior long after their usefulness to the organism has become anachronistic. No easy assessment of what is defined as culture is available, but it can be understood best by Kluckhohn's approach to the problem. According to him, there are five questions that man, regardless of the level of sophistication of his culture, asks himself, whether he is aware of it or not. These questions can be answered within a spectrum, and while each society may relate to the entire spectrum, it is the inordinate emphasis that is placed on one of these answers that determines the society's value system, its child rearing practices, its behavior, and may I add its treatment of the aged. A brief examination of one or two of these questions may illustrate my point.

What is man's relationship to time? Which of the three time orientations, past, present, or future, does he value most? There is, of course, no question that we as Americans value the future. Our future-mindedness makes planners of us all. Nothing is left to chance, not even a spontaneous good time. We are so busy planning for the future that, when the future catches up with us and becomes the present, we cannot enjoy it because we are again busy planning for the future. As a result, as Americans, we cannot have a good time and enjoy the present. We seldom sit anywhere without feeling that we should be somewhere else. How does this affect older Americans? Not only are they people without a future and hence not ones to invest in, but having incorporated the valued time orientation, they, the only group in our society meant to do so, are incapable of enjoying the present, and the hope for a better future is a mirage in the twilight of life.

Another question: what type of personality is valued most? The "being" — the individual who is mainly concerned with feelings, impulses, and desires of the moment; the "being in becoming" — most interested in inner development and the fullest realization of aspects of personality; or the "doing" — the one principally concerned with action, achievement, and getting things done? It is not too difficult to recognize ourselves in this configuration. We are the doers. While the Mexican mother, valuing the "being" orientation, may happily enjoy her child from day to day, the American mother is too often concerned with his progress. His achievements are a measure of her competence as a mother, an efficient manager, and a force in the community. Doing, too, must have a by-product discernable to one of our senses. We unconsciously depreciate the contemplative aspects of life. One does nothing when one reads or thinks.

Here again we can readily recognize the impact of such an orientation on the aging organism. The old have stopped doing, are alien in our eyes and depreciated in their own. Nor have they prepared their lives for a contemplative existence. The effects are often quite devastating, resulting frequently in restlessness and purposeless agitation.

My hope is that I have succeeded in acquainting the reader with the thinking of a clinician in his attempts to understand a very complex problem. Implicit in all that I have said lurk some therapeutic maneuvers so necessary to alleviate the suffering of our aged population.

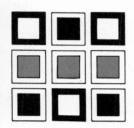

Review of Proceedings:
Directions for Future Research

Ewald W. Busse, M.D.

Department of Psychiatry, Duke University College
of Medicine, Durham, North Carolina

In reviewing the proceedings of this meeting, I would prefer not to touch upon the individual papers but rather to confine my remarks to two separate areas of concern and interest. First, I would like to mention the things I believe were scientifically exciting. Second, I will want to touch upon aspects of the aging brain that I felt were omitted from this excellent program.

Early in the proceedings we were reminded of the possible correlation between the sequential onset of developmental processes to the appearance of aging changes; that is, are the developmental processes that appear early in life the first to undergo age changes, and does the speed of the developmental process correlate with the subsequent speed of decline? If we had a better understanding of this parallelism in aging and development, it is conceivable that it would add considerably to our knowledge.

The second item of great interest to me is the concept of stress and how stress affects the individual. I believe it is important to differentiate types of stress, particularly those that are characterized by an overload of stimuli or hostile impulses, as contrasted to the type of stress that results from a deprivation of stimuli critical to maintaining a physiological balance and mental functioning. In my opinion it is highly likely that older people suffer more losses from deprivation stress than from traumatic stress. This thought permits me to progress to a related concern: in my opinion, elderly people can be identified who do not accommodate to their physiological change; that is, they expect to react as they did at an earlier age, and when they recognize that they have changed and do not accommodate, this accentuates their anxiety. They have not accommodated effectively to the aging process. Hence there is a greater loss of efficiency than is found in those who do accommodate to aging changes free of anxiety.

217

Another interesting subject relates to the frequency of senile plaques associated with Down's syndrome. It is my impression that this offers an opportunity to determine whether senile plaques, as they occur in a broad spectrum of individuals, are actually the end-result of a common pathological process or whether the senile plaque is similar but the end-result of several different processes.

An area that demands closer attention is the deficiency in our diagnostic system that seriously impairs clinical investigation. I believe, for example, that we should attempt to distinguish brain changes that are the result of intrinsic vascular changes from brain changes that are attributable to external cardiovascular disease. The latter could easily account for the failure to detect vascular changes within the brain when the deterioration appears to be related to a decrease in cerebral blood flow. Somewhat similarly, it is my belief that more attention should be given to age changes associated with autoregulation by the brain of its blood flow. It is not only possible that autoregulation becomes less efficient, but it is possible also that it moves toward paradoxical responses.

I am disappointed that more attention was not given to the dispute regarding Alzheimer's disease and senile dementia. Apparently there is unanimity in this symposium that so-called Alzheimer's disease is an early form of senile dementia. However, all of us are quite aware that the literature, particularly the European literature, indicates the persistence of considerable difference of opinion and that contradicting data have been presented. Perhaps in a future symposium this complex subject can be explored in depth.

I was also a little disappointed that the complicated but important subject of autoimmunity was given little attention. There is little doubt that the elderly person loses his capacity to mobilize his immune responses to infection, yet at the same time there is a rapid increase in the frequency of autoimmune diseases. I hope that some of these subjects will be pursued in a follow-up symposium.

Questions for the Future

As for the future of research funding and research training in the field of aging, there are a number of questions that haunt me. For example, in spite of an increase in our training efforts, have we really succeeded in attracting a sufficient number of competent investigators to the field of aging? If we have not, why not? I have already expressed the opinion that our growth has not been satisfactory, and it is conceivable that this is a reflection of the lack of concern with aging and the aged which seems to permeate most of our society.

Those interested in the clinical care of the elderly are constantly confronted with the lack of interest on the part of professionals and nonprofessionals in providing good care for the elderly. I recognize that there are a number of people at this conference who have worked very diligently in the past few years to improve this situation. Dr. Birren, while at the National Institute of Child Health and Human Development, strove with all his effort to improve this situation, and he has continued to do so. Other leaders in the field of gerontology, among them Drs. Bernard Strehler, Carl Eisdorfer, and F. Marrott Sinex, have worked diligently and with some success to increase the funding of research and research training. But I do not believe that the time and effort that they have put into this work is really reflected in the results. We must continue, therefore, to identify the resistances and counterforces that make our progress so slow.

Dr. Maurice Van Allen mentioned his observation that members of the United States Senate seem to be increasingly interested in the field of aging and hinted that this is true because the Senators are approaching old age or are actually in the latter years of their lives. Unfortunately, in my opinion, this interest is not evident in their actions, as, all too often when the chips are down, they and others in leadership position do not seem committed to improving the lot of the elderly. They justify this lack of commitment by saying that the field of aging does not have enough of what they call "clout." Political expedience seems to take precedence over social and scientific needs. Again this year we are facing the fact that a considerable amount of money that should be available for research in the field of aging has not yet been released for allocation by government officials. It is obvious that if we are to contribute to the understanding of the aging process and the improvement of the lives of older people, we will have to participate in the political process and educate the decision-makers so that a reasonable amount of our resources is allocated to a better understanding of aging and the brain.

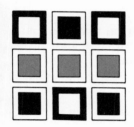

Toward an Interdisciplinary Approach

James E. Birren, Ph.D.

Gerontology Center, University of Southern
California, Los Angeles, California

An overview of some fifteen comprehensive papers is difficult. It struck me during the course of the meetings that the problems we are dealing with in aging of the brain are very large issues, and that there is a life span of these natural problems that is much longer than any one of our individual life spans. Some of these problems, therefore, are more suited for institutional development than the development during individual careers. In fact, the productive life span of an individual researcher seems quite short in relation to these problems.

Take the issue of the pigment lipofuscin. These cellular deposits in old brain cells probably have been known for a hundred years. We still do not know whether lipofuscin is good or bad in the cell; we do not know its origin, and we are not sure about its physiological or functional significance. I hope we can make more rapid progress in understanding the aging nervous system; perhaps the investment needs to be greater than the laboratory and skills of any one individual and even any one institution. I believe also that approaching the problems by single disciplines may be a mistake. When we look at something like Alzheimer's disease, which has been a focus of our attention, it seems to me it is a problem of such magnitude that we ought to use a health research team concept in which the neuroanatomists, neurologists, psychiatrists, psychologists, and others will adopt a problem orientation. It would seem that working on senile dementia within departments, as we have done, has not yielded much progress. I do not mean to sound overly critical, but we have not, in fact, made much of a dent in these problems in the last twenty-five years. So perhaps in settings like this, the Texas Research Institute of Mental Sciences, there may be better opportunities to conceive and put into operation research on the aging brain and such deteriorative diseases of late life as Alzheimer's disease. This may yield more success because, with the neuroanatomists feeling that the physiologists and the neurochemists are looking over their shoulders, they will begin to consider how

221

to relate some of the structural changes to function.

In this process of interdisciplinary exchange, I noticed that we all use metaphors to allude to the landmarks in our understanding, and that we tend to reify these metaphors. Until we come to a meeting like this, we are not really aware how much we have reified them. Our metaphors become real things in our minds. With apologies to Dr. Foley, we have shown within the disciplines a deification of the reification. In the process of penetrating some of this reification, I believe we were excessively polite, perhaps because this was the first interdisciplinary meeting on this topic. We ought to learn something from the young students because they are pushing us to ask harder, more penetrating questions than we allow ourselves in a meeting of this sort. We must learn to ask penetrating questions in a way that is supportive rather than destructive. That takes a little art; some of the younger people here in the sciences and professions know that art better than we do.

I judge that most progress has been made in the past interval in understanding the physiology of the whole brain. I sense that results of metabolic studies and blood flow studies offer us data that are useful in relating to other issues. With apologies to my own field, psychology, and also to neuroanatomy, I could not integrate the data very well yet, but in the physiology of the whole brain we are beginning to do so. In this perspective, I expect more contributions in the next few years from physiology than I do from some of the other disciplines, except perhaps in those institutions where research may be organized with a problem or health team concept.

Some new techniques are obviously available to us and they are being reported, but I am not certain how soon the data yielded by these new techniques will be relatable to the aging brain. Take the issue of localization of brain function in psychology. I do not believe psychologists have really put their hands to the task of understanding the deficits of old people. They could have done a much better job in the last ten years than has been done, because I do not believe we can screen individuals and localize specific deficits the way we should at this point. We should look, perhaps, beyond the EEG to the work on sensory evoked potentials and contingent negative variation. Some of these techniques will help us to understand the electrophysiology of the aging brain and to bridge the behavioral and physiological data; that is where the gains are going to come in the near future.

It is difficult to stop short of looking into some of the detailed contributions that have been made at this conference, although I have done it because I am impressed by the magnitude of the issues we face.

This symposium began with the charge to identify the critical issues in mental health and aging, to define the problems more clearly, and to suggest solutions, stimulate research, clarify needs, and to rank problems in some priority fashion. We have not completed this job and I would suggest that this should be but the first of a series of conferences on the same subject matter, although future conferences might be more limited in scope, now that we have a perspective on the total field. We have reached sufficient maturity in our interdisciplinary attitudes to begin to tackle through research the problems of aging and the brain, problems that transcend many disciplines. I think this field has needed some paternity, if not grand-paternity, and perhaps the Texas Research Institute of Mental Sciences could exercise this paternity. The scope of the issues requires that some institutions organize an interdisciplinary program of research on aging of the brain, a program that will not only lead to an understanding of some of the basic processes, but also facilitate training and diagnosis and treatment.

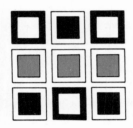

Epilogue

Charles M. Gaitz, M.D.

Gerontology Research Section
Texas Research Institute of Mental Sciences
Houston, Texas

Experts in a number of disciplines concerned with aging and the brain met and had an opportunity to exchange information and ideas. Interesting papers were presented, the discussion was lively and, on the whole, it seemed clear that most participants thought the three-day symposium had been a valuable experience.

The central question remains, have we done justice to the plight of the elderly? Obviously we have not. Many questions have no answers yet, and others are answered without unanimity. Conceptualization of normal and abnormal aging requires more attention. Treatment modalities need further evaluation, and treatment is still more often pragmatic than based on solid scientific knowledge. The authors of the preceding chapters have given us a picture of the current status of knowledge about aging and the brain, but each has acknowledged gaps in understanding, the need for further research and, deliberately or not, has given us some directions for future progress. Some have taken a rather pessimistic view; others feel that we are taking small but positive steps toward a better understanding of brain function, especially as it relates to aging and associated processes.

Shortly after this symposium was held, Dr. Seymour S. Kety, professor of psychiatry at Harvard Medical School, was quoted (*Hospital Tribune*, November 29, 1971) as expressing little hope that the behavioral output of the brain can be explained in molecular terms. It was his opinion that "the information storage, the comparisons, and discriminations involved in a human decision are distributed over millions of neurons, making its description or comprehension at that level extremely remote." Nevertheless, he thought that drugs, though they have inherent limitations, may be quite valuable in influencing learning and memory processes. He expressed the belief that where learning or

225

some of its components—like attention, memory, or performance—are impaired by disease, metabolic defect, or nutritional inadequacy, continued research would be able to specify the deficits, so that the biological causes might be corrected. He pointed out that impaired cerebral circulation accounts for a substantial segment of the senile dementias, and that it is not unreasonable to expect arteriosclerosis of the brain as well as the heart eventually to yield to biochemically based comprehension and therapy.

To emphasize the need for further studies is redundant. What perhaps should be emphasized is the need for more investigations involving the approaches of several professional disciplines, not only those represented at the symposium, but also those in sociologic and economic planning. It was impossible to establish a hierarchy of specific areas to be studied. All are important, and no one can predict the field or area most likely to lead to significant insights and better treatment.

Becoming "senile" is perhaps the most frightening of all prospects for persons in the middle and late years of their lives. Yet researchers have shown relatively little interest in pursuing studies in this area. Possibly this resistance and apathy originates in hopeless attitudes toward aging and senility. It seems quite likely, though, that we are now at a stage when the technology is available, or could be available, to assist investigators in resolving some very complex but fascinating problems. We must find ways to interest more people, researchers in many disciplines, to apply themselves to the processes of aging, and specifically to those related to brain function. These studies need not be confined to elderly subjects; they should be viewed as studies of the full panorama of human existence. Seen in this way, research aimed at elevating the potentialities of each stage of living will hold greater attraction and reward for the investigator and the investigated.

Index

Acetylcholine, 150
Acetylcholinesterase in brain, 44
Acoustic neuroma, 158
Actihaemyl, 205
Aging
  cognitive change, 5
  model, 8
  neurochemistry, 41
  neuropsychological assessment, 29
Alzheimer's disease, 48, 65, 159, 185,
  206, 218
  associated with Down's syndrome,
    68, 75
  morphological change, 89
  protein synthesis, 94
  substructure, 106
Amitriptyline, 199
Amnesia
  parietal lobe symptom, 16
Amobarbital, 196, 200
Amphetamine, 194
Amyloid, 65, 99
  amyloidosis, 68, 173
Anger, 189
Anosognosia, 154
Aortocranial arteriography, 138
Aphasia, 159
Arteriosclerotic brain disease, 65, 81,
  119, 136
Arteriosclerotic dementia, 21, 135
  distribution, 22
  treated with lipotropic enzymes,
    205

Arteriovenous oxygen difference
  in aging, 127
  in brain atrophy and Wernicke-Korsakoff
    syndrome, 129
Atheroma, 205
Atropine, 150
Autoimmunity, 218
Autonomic nervous system in aging, 145, 149

Basal ganglia
  Creutzfeldt-Jacob disease, 76
  lesion, 155
Behavior
  diagnosis, 154, 209
  exploitative-manipulative, 184
  functional groups, 155
  pattern, 212
  relationship to brain, 30
    cultural pattern, 214
    sensory input, 165
B-glucuronidase, 205
Blood pressure
  in aging, 147
  in organic brain disease, 124
Brain
  aging process, 179
  composition, 42
  DNA, 43, 44
  neutral fat, 43
  normal aging, 81
  oxygen consumption, 43
  phosphorus content, 43
  subcellular components, 46